Essentials of Death Reporting and Death Certification

Practical Applications for the Clinical Practitioner

Erica J. Armstrong MD

Acknowledgements

The Author would like to thank Forensic Photographers Kate Snyder, Amy Koons, and Jason Bielinski for the acquisition and formatting of the digital images included in this text. The Author would also like to thank Mr. Joe Stopak BS, D-ABMDI, Manager of Investigation and Morgue Operations at CCMEO and custodian of "Coroner Amendment" death certificates.

Printed in the United States of America

First printing, 2017

ISBN-13: 978-0-9985334-0-7 (soft cover)

Dedication

To all of the dedicated professionals and public servants who strive daily to improve and maintain the Nation's health, safety, and well-being.

TABLE OF CONTENTS

About the Author

Dr. Erica J. Armstrong is a board certified Forensic Pathologist and medicolegal consultant currently practicing in Cleveland, Ohio, with over 16 years of experience.

Dr. Armstrong earned her Bachelor of Science degree with a major in Biology-Premed from Notre Dame College of Ohio. She earned her Doctor of Medicine degree from Case Western Reserve University School of Medicine (CWRU-SOM). She completed her residency training in combined anatomic and clinical pathology at University Hospitals of Cleveland where she served as Chief Resident in Pathology. Following residency, she completed 2 years of fellowship training in Forensic Pathology at the Cuyahoga County Coroner's Office (CCCO) where she received mentorship from the well-respected and longtime Coroner Dr. Elizabeth Balraj and the late Chief Deputy Coroner, Dr. Robert Challener. She remained on staff as Deputy Coroner and subsequently Deputy Medical Examiner when CCCO became a medical examiner's office in 2011 which is now known as the Cuyahoga County Medical Examiner's Office-Cuyahoga County Regional Forensic Science Laboratory (CCMEO-CCRFSL).

To date, she has performed more than 3,400 forensic autopsies with cause and manner of death determination and death certification. These include complex natural, accidental, homicidal and suicidal deaths. She is qualified as an expert witness in forensic pathology and has given expert courtroom and deposition testimony on numerous occasions.

In addition to her daily duties, Dr. Armstrong provides information and mentorship regarding the practice of forensic pathology, for the lay community, allied health community, law enforcement community, legal community, medical students and doctors-in-training. For nearly a decade as Director of Medical Education at CCMEO-CCRFSL she has run and participated in the year-round student/resident elective rotation program provided to medical students, physician assistant students, and both clinical and pathology residents. She has greatly improved the learning experience of participants of the program by developing and administering testing and teaching materials, evaluating performance, and assigning projects. All educational and testing materials cover concepts and definitions of death reporting, cause and manner of death, and death certification in addition to core topics in forensic pathology. Students in the allied health, criminal justice, paralegal, and undergraduate biological sciences are provided introduction to and review of gross anatomy with clinicopathologic correlation by way of autopsy demonstration classes for which she additionally directs. She holds clinical teaching appointments at both medical and osteopathic schools. She is the Activity Director of the CCMEO Lecture Series, a weekly educational activity with presentations from in-house staff and outside guest speakers covering clinical medicine, forensic science, and forensic pathology topics.

Dr. Armstrong has authored numerous journal articles and a single textbook on topics in anatomic, clinical, and forensic pathology afforded by medical training, practice experience, mentors, and numerous interactions with those in clinical medicine. *Essentials of Death Reporting and Death Certification-Practical Applications for the Clinical Practitioner* represents the fruits of those invaluable experiences.

CHAPTER 1

INTRODUCTION

Death Certification: A Professional Duty and Final Courtesy to Your Patient

The practice of medicine strives to prevent and treat disease while prolonging and improving the quality of life. The death of a patient is always untimely, whether expected or not. It may be difficult for the clinician (physician, physician assistant, nurse practitioner, or other caretakers) to accept this inevitability and eventuality, especially after the best of clinical efforts. When faced with the loss of a patient, the clinician must master the ability to explain to family members in understandable terms why their loved one has died. It is also the professional duty of the clinician to provide an official statement of the cause of death by way of the death certificate.

Clinicians-in-training receive very little in the way of instruction in death reporting and death certification which generally occurs during the earliest part of their training, soon to be forgotten due to the mountain of clinical material and procedures that must be mastered over the ensuing years of training. Some clinicians may feel apprehensive about certifying a death--that putting the wrong cause of death on the death certificate may trigger a lawsuit or some other form of retribution. There may be concern that listing a particular cause of death may stigmatize or embarrass the family, preclude the processing of an insurance claim, or raise legal issues that delay the settling of an estate. The occasional need to certify a death may even seem more a nuisance rather than a professional duty, like rendering a clinical diagnosis or prescribing a therapeutic regimen. Although there is no real legal consequence for a clinician who repeatedly fails to complete a death certificate in a timely manner, he or she can be reported to the state licensing board triggering an investigation and possible formal disciplinary action, which then becomes public record. Families may express their dissatisfaction through social media and internet-based survey forums or through direct communication with hospital administration or the affiliated ombudsman.

The notion that death certification is unimportant having no effects could not be further from the truth. An important general benefit of proper death certification is the optimization of health care via prevention of morbidity and mortality. The consequences of delayed completion a death certificate are wide ranging and most importantly include extreme emotional and financial hardship to the family. One needs only to imagine the hardships that could result from the inability to settle a family estate, to acquire social security benefits, or to acquire life insurance funds. Family members may be forced to drain personal savings or investment accounts in order to make ends meet or pay funeral costs while waiting for the completed death certificate, uprooting their sense of financial security. Those families not fortunate enough to have savings or investments and/or their deceased loved one was the sole or primary earner, are without financial alternatives. The inability to pay creditors may prompt bankruptcy filing or precipitate financial ruin. Without the death certificate families are also unable to:

- Bury or cremate their loved one
- Access bank accounts and retirement/pension plan funds
- Close the decedent's bank, credit card, or utility accounts
- Transfer living legal next-of-kin, beneficiary, or administrator's name to decedent's bank, credit card, or utility accounts
- Make mortgage and utility bill payments or pay medical bills incurred after a loved one's prolonged terminal hospitalization
- Continue the grieving process

These hardships added with the grief of losing a loved one are only compounded by the absence of closure left by a delayed or incomplete death certificate. Bereaved families left with uncertainty regarding the death of their loved one are more apt to suspect substandard medical care and seek legal advice up to and including filing a lawsuit against any or all members of the clinical care team for malpractice or wrongful death.

The role that the forensic pathologist plays in the spectrum of the practice of medicine is often underappreciated or unknown altogether. To a degree, this is understandable since medical students and medical residents generally do not receive sufficient amounts of required exposure to and instruction in anatomic pathology, an important conduit to the subspecialty of forensic pathology. As the rate of hospital autopsies continues to decline and less emphasis is placed on gross and microscopic pathology, this problem will only worsen. The forensic pathologist working in the medical examiner's or coroner's office is directly involved in the investigation of sudden, unexplained and unnatural deaths. This requires application of knowledge of clinical medicine, laboratory medicine, forensic science, and pathology for the resolution of deaths, often within the context of law. This can include the investigation of therapy-associated deaths arising from misdiagnosis, delayed diagnosis, failure to diagnose, or medical error. The forensic pathologist, having reviewed the clinical records and performed the autopsy, may later provide expert medical testimony by way of deposition or court trial as to the autopsy findings and the cause and manner of death, relative to a claim filed on behalf of the decedent. Forensic pathologists also certify deaths on a very regular basis and as such are a rich source of information on the "how to" of death certification.

CHAPTER 2

DEATH INVESTIGATIVE SYSTEMS

2.1 Death Monitoring in the United States

In the United States, a great amount of statistical information is derived from the classification of deaths arising from a multitude of causes, providing researchers and clinical practitioners with foundational information upon which to improve medical diagnosis and enhance medical care. The International Classification of Diseases, currently in its tenth edition (ICD-10), was created by the World Health Organization (WHO) as a medical classification system not only for disease and injury of the living but also disease and injury causing death [1]. The classification of a given death is derived directly from the information provided in the cause-of-death statement on the death certificate. The more specific the information contained in the cause-of-death statement, the more accurate the classification of the death and therefore the statistical data regarding morbidity and mortality. For example, the cause-of-death statement "Hypertensive cardiovascular disease" can be coded and classified into the category associated with diseases of the circulatory system, whereas "Cardiac arrest" has no etiologic specificity as to what led to the arrest (heart-related versus related to some other organ system versus related to some type of injury or intoxication), and thus cannot be further classified.

Offices involved with medicolegal death investigation led by medical examiners and coroners generate a wealth of information beyond causes of death that is of vital interest to many federal departments and agencies charged with the surveillance of disease, injury, product safety and national security. These include the Centers for Disease Control and Prevention-National Center of Health Statistics (CDC-NCHS), the National Institutes of Health (NIH), the Food and Drug Administration (FDA), the Consumer Product Safety Commission (CPSC), the United States Department of Homeland Security, and many others.

The cause-of-death information derived from the death certificate is recorded and tracked locally by city health departments and vital statistics bureaus, on the state level, nationally and internationally. The CDC-NCHS provides the national function for the United States providing our Country's health information beginning with the systematic collection of standardized mortality statistics directed by the National Vital Statistics System (NVSS), a part of the CDC-NCHS. As a signatory of WHO, the Nation's health data is in turn utilized for international comparisons and ranking.

Physician medical examiners and coroners are involved on a routine basis in the certification of deaths due to disease, injury, and poisoning. Clinicians including physicians, nurse practitioners, and physician assistants, while not involved with certification of deaths due to injury and poisoning, nevertheless provide information via ICD coding regarding patients who have sustained injury or poisoning with treatment and discharge from medical facilities. Cause-of-death information on death certificates and clinical diagnostic information from medical records are given ICD codes which facilitate classification. Important information and trends regarding various environmental and health hazards are extracted from statistical and epidemiological analyses of coded disease data which in turn ultimately give rise to safety bulletins and press releases that inform healthcare providers and the general public.

A number of online resources allow interactive and searchable review of health trends and the impact of diseases, injuries, and deaths. Many include periodic reports available in a downloadable format or for purchase. Yearly death data including the total deaths, the death rate, life expectancy, age-specific death rates, the leading cause of death, and the infant mortality rate are reported in the National Vital Statistics Report [2]. The National Violent Death Reporting System (NVDRS) collects incident-specific data from death certificates, medical examiner and coroner reports, law enforcement reports, and crime laboratories and make those data accessible via the user friendly and interactive website provided by the CDC's Web-based Injury Statistics Query and Reporting System (WISQARS) [3]. The National Safety Council is an additional online source of information regarding preventable injuries and deaths arising in the workplace, in the home, and in communities [4]. Other surveillance programs with a focus on public health and safety also utilize information contained in law enforcement investigative reports, medical records and death certificates with just a select few presented here:

- Drug Abuse Warning Network-DAWN www.samhsa.gov (created by the Substance Abuse and Mental Health Services Administration-SAMHSA with information on emergency room visits and deaths resulting from abuse and misuse of drugs and substances)
- Food and Drug Administration (FDA) Medical Products Program-MedWatch www.fda.gov/medwatch (information on adverse events or deaths resulting from medical devices and medication errors)
- Fatality Analysis Reporting System-FARS www.nhtsa.gov/FARS (division of the National Highway Traffic Safety Administration-NHTSA with information on factors leading to fatal motor vehicle crashes)
- National Poison Data System-NPDS www.aapcc.org (created under the American Association of Poison Control Centers with annual reporting on trends in exposures to various substances published in the Clinical Toxicology journal)
- Medical Examiners and Coroners Alert Project (MECAP) www.cpsc.gov/en/Research--Statistics/MECAP? (created under the US Consumer Product Safety Commission; collects information reported by medical examiner/coroner offices and from death certificates regarding deaths associated with consumer products with yearly publication of data and newsletters)
- Morbidity and Mortality Weekly Report (MMWR) www.cdc.gov/mmwr/index.html (regular series of reports and articles regarding public health information and recommendations from state-based morbidity and mortality information, produced by the CDC)

According to the CDC, drug overdose is the leading cause of injury death in the United States for ages 25 to 64 having surpassed motor vehicle traffic crashes. The death rate has more than doubled during 1999-2013, from 6.0 per 100,000 population in 1999 to 13.8 in 2013 [5]. Over the recent years particularly, an epidemic of heroin and prescription pain medication misuse and abuse has gripped the nation and many other parts of the world with deadly consequences and with no signs of abating. Patients with chronic pain conditions or those recovering from injuries and surgical and dental procedures make up a significant part of this vulnerable population. Prescription medications such as hydrocodone, oxycodone, oxymorphone, methadone, benzodiazepines, stimulants, and muscle relaxants have been identified in clinical and postmortem laboratory testing. More recently, fentanyl and derivatives like acetyl fentanyl, clandestinely manufactured and sold in lieu of or mixed with heroin, have also contributed to spikes in emergency department visits and deaths [6]. The combination of "doctor shopping" for prescriptions for nonmedical use and resale added with overprescribing by clinicians has been identified to correlate positively to the sharp rise in hospital visits and deaths. In response to the staggering statistics and as an effort to combat the prescription overdose epidemic by providing awareness to the public and clinical practitioners, a number of states have developed prescription monitoring programs to identify controlled substance prescribing patterns and misuse/abuse behaviors. These programs extract data from information provided in medical records and medical examiner/coroner-generated reports and death certificates. Since 2012, these data have been submitted for analysis to the Prescription Behavior Surveillance System (PBSS) funded by the CDC and FDA. Surveillance summaries on controlled substance prescribing patterns are published in the MMWR.

Aside from the established reporting and surveillance systems, an abundance of information regarding cause, mechanism, and manner of many types of deaths, often with pathological correlation to clinical presentation, can be found in the forensic pathology literature. Reports of disease and injury manifestations often presenting as sudden and unexpected death appear in the clinical medicine and dentistry literature as well. Below is a select list of well-established, peer-reviewed general pathology and forensic science/pathology journals:

- Academic Forensic Pathology (www.afpjournal.com)
- American Journal of Forensic Medicine and Pathology (journals.lww.com/amjforensicmedicine/Pages/default.aspx)
- Archives of Pathology and Laboratory Medicine (www.archivesofpathology.org)
- Forensic Science International (www.journals.elsevier.com/forensic-science-international)
- Forensic Science, Medicine, and Pathology (www.springer.com/medicine/pathology/journal/12024)
- Journal of Forensic and Legal Medicine (www.journals.elsevier.com/journal-of-forensic-and-legal-medicine)
- Journal of Forensic Sciences (onlinelibrary.wiley.com/journal/10.1111/%28ISSN%291556-4029)

- Legal Medicine (www.journals.elsevier.com/legal-medicine)
- Medicine, Science, and the Law (msl.sagepub.com)

2.2 Death Investigative Systems in the United States

Death investigation in the United States has its origins in England, based on the 1194 Articles of Eyre, established under Richard the Lionhearted, which provided for the keepers of the pleas of the crown, the origin of the word "coroner". The coroner's official duty was to protect the king's financial interest in criminal proceedings and to investigate sudden and unnatural deaths. The office of the coroner was later incorporated into the United States governmental structure by the early North American settlers [7]. The realization that a medical professional was needed to participate in or oversee death investigation began with the enactment of laws in Maryland, Massachusetts, and New York, from 1860-1902. This included the requirement of a coroner physician or appointment of physicians by coroners to participate in death investigation as a medical examiner. The first medical examiner-type system operated in the state of New York in the early 1900's and with subsequent institution across the country as more individuals became trained. The 1954 Model Postmortem Examinations Act provided a framework upon which the concept and operation of a comprehensive medical examiner system could be built but to date has not been widely or fully instituted for a number of reasons including issues and difficulties with politics, legislation, geography, and infrastructure and acquiring trained personnel [8]. Over time, a gradual shift from coroner to medical examiner systems has occurred in the United States, albeit at a slow pace, with recent such conversion occurring in Cuyahoga County of Ohio after an amendment in the state's charter which took effect in 2011.

The monitoring of our Nation's health is inextricably linked to the outcomes of medicolegal death investigation, in which the circumstances surrounding sudden, unexpected, and unnatural deaths are carefully reviewed and their cause(s) elucidated. Under the provision of state law, with slight variations between the States, rules regarding medicolegal death investigation and the individuals involved are put forth. The results of death investigation provide a vast database for epidemiological research used for public health surveillance and for the improvement and promotion of public health and welfare through reduction of morbidity and mortality.

In the United States, the investigation of sudden, unexpected, unexplained, and unnatural deaths is an official proceeding mostly conducted by either a **medical examiner** or **coroner**, within a certain geographical location or jurisdiction: a state, a region or district within a state (multiple counties), a county, or a city as outlined in the statutes. Approximately 3,145 county-equivalent jurisdictions, 25 state-wide systems, and 95 regional or district systems containing multiple counties exist in the United States [9,10,11]. The majority of the United States population resides in areas served by a medical examiner, which tend to be in more densely populated locations. That leaves the remaining population, often in smaller and more rural locations, served by coroners. In some rural counties within the state of Texas, the Justice of the Peace performs coroner duties including pronouncement of death and death certification. The majority (approximately 80%) of medical examiner/coroner offices are county coroner's offices.

Each system serving a particular jurisdiction has in charge of it a medical examiner or a coroner charged with investigating sudden, unexpected and unnatural deaths or deaths known or suspected to be the result of injury, poisoning/intoxication, or violence, for the purpose of determining the cause and manner of death. A **medical examiner** is almost always a physician (M.D. or D.O.), usually a pathologist, and often a forensic pathologist. The (chief) medical examiner is appointed by the governmental entity of the jurisdiction (i.e. the county executive). A **coroner** is usually elected by the voters and in most states, is not required to be a physician (except OH, LA, ND, and KS), and with no special requirements other than to be eligible to vote. Moreover, interstate variation as to the professional and educational requirements for both medical examiners and coroners exists. The sheriff or a funeral director often fulfills the role of a non-physician coroner in some locales. Many physician coroners practice in a variety of non-pathology specialties such as emergency medicine, family medicine, and radiology. Physician coroners may also be forensic pathologists. Both non-physician and physician coroners employ, directly or contractually, forensically trained pathologists (coroner's pathologists) to perform autopsies and assist with death investigation. Both medical examiners and coroners additionally utilize the expertise of forensic scientists and medicolegal death investigators to assist them with laboratory testing and death scene investigation.

Death investigative systems designated as medical examiner or coroner's offices may operate as stand-alone forensic scientific centers or be linked administratively to local government, the sheriff's department, a hospital system, or the health department. Increasingly, private forensic pathology practices are in operation that provide comprehensive services on a contractual basis to local governments and/or provide à la carte services to attorneys and the public. Many well-funded and well-run offices contain on-site laboratories involved in the performance of autopsies and the handling and testing of evidence, drugs and chemicals, and biological samples. The results that are generated from autopsies and forensic scientific testing are applied to the settlement of criminal and civil cases which is central to the overall practice of forensic science and forensic pathology. This important work is not possible without specially trained professionals including but not limited to forensic pathologists, pathologist assistants, forensic trace evidence and DNA scientists, forensic toxicologists and chemists, firearms and tool mark analysts, fingerprint analysts, forensic anthropologists, forensic odontologists, forensic photographers, and medicolegal death investigators. In particular is the **medicolegal death investigator** who may have a range of prior experience and training and/ or have completed training with certification by the American Board of Medicolegal Death Investigators (ABMDI). These individuals are the "front line" representatives of the medical examiner or coroner's office responsible for receiving the initial call of the report of death, frequently from medical facilities. Many offices also generate their own yearly statistical reports detailing the results of investigation of jurisdictional deaths including results of laboratory testing.

Organizations such as the National Association of Medical Examiners (NAME), American Academy of Forensic Sciences (AAFS), International Association of Coroners and Medical Examiners (IACME), the American Board of Medicolegal Death Investigators (ABMDI), the American Society of Crime Laboratory Directors/Laboratory Accreditation Board (ASCLD/LAB), American Association of Blood Banks (AABB), American Board of Forensic Toxicology (ABFT), and a number of in-state coroner and medical examiner associations publish, practice or promote standards and recommendations for high-quality forensic medicolegal death investigation within death investigation systems. Moreover, NAME, ASCLD/LAB, AABB, and ABFT are accreditation agencies that by application of their rigorous inspection programs, ensure that offices involved in medicolegal death investigation maintain high standards of practice and reporting. All of the above organizations each have comprehensive and educational websites and relevant links.

References

1. International Classifications of Diseases (ICD). World Health Organization. Available at: www.who.int/classifications/icd/en .

2. Kochanek KD and Murphy SL. Deaths: final data for 2011. *Natl Vital Stat Rep.* 2015; 63(3):1-120. Available on www.cdc.gov.

3. Web-based Injury Statistics Query and Reporting System (WISQARS). Available at: www.cdc/gov/injury/wisqars.

4. National Safety Council. Available at: www.nsc.org .

5. www.cdc.gov/drugoverdose/data/overdose/html . Accessed 12/27/2015.

6. Rudd RA, Aleshire JD, Zibbell JE, and Gladden RM. Increase in drug and opioid overdose deaths-United States, 2000-2014. January 1, 2016. *MMWR*. 64(50):1378-82.

7. Fisher RS, Platt MS. History of forensic pathology and related laboratory sciences. In*: Spitz and Fisher's Medicolegal Investigation of Death: Guidelines for the Application of Pathology to Crime Investigation. 4th edition.* Springfield Illinois: CC Thomas Publishers.

8. Hanzlick R. The conversion of coroner systems to medical examiner systems in the United States: A lull in action. *Am J Forensic Med Pathol.* 2007;28(4):279-283.

9. Hanzlick R L. Medical examiners, coroners, and public health-A review and update. *Arch Pathol Lab Med.* 2006;130(9):1274-82.

10. Hanzlick, R L. A perspective on medicolegal death investigation in the United States:2013. *Acad Forensic Pathol.* 2014;4(1):2-9.

11. Gill J R. State medical examiner systems, 2013: Staffing, autopsies, strengths, limitations, and needs. *Acad Forensic Pathol.* 2014;4(1):24-31.

CHAPTER 3

REPORTING A DEATH TO THE MEDICAL EXAMINER OR CORONER

3.1 General Considerations

Certain deaths fall under the jurisdiction of the Medical Examiner or Coroner (ME/C) as outlined by the laws of each state. These laws delineate the types of deaths reportable and the requirements of the ME/C including the notification of the legal next-of-kin, record keeping, and the provision of laboratory services [1]. In 2004, approximately 1 million US deaths or 30-40% of all deaths were referred to ME/C offices with 50% of those accepted and investigated by those offices for determination of cause and manner of death [2].

In general, jurisdictional deaths are sudden, unexpected, unexplained, unnatural, or violent deaths and deaths unattended by a physician inclusive of the **attending physician**. Importantly, *any* physician that has previously evaluated or treated the decedent in the office, hospital, or home setting, or has written prescriptions for that individual, by definition is considered as the attending physician or simply the **treating physician** and need not be physically present at the time of the patient's death. The physician of record including not only the attending physician but also the **pronouncing physician** will have knowledge of or access to some facet of the medical history that could have importance and relevance to the cause of death. Physicians practicing in the **primary care specialties** (emergency medicine, internal medicine, family medicine, pediatrics, geriatrics, general obstetrics/gynecology, and general surgery) would especially qualify as having firsthand knowledge of a patient's medical history. Psychiatrists could also be included in this group and the sudden death in a psychiatric patient, who has known, documented chronic natural disease with lethal potential and was otherwise not exhibiting psychosis of suicidal symptomatology prior to death, would not necessarily come under the jurisdiction of the ME/C. However, the sudden death of a psychiatric patient with recent psychosis, suicidal ideation or attempt, or recent hospitalization for treatment of a psychiatric condition, is a reportable death and would likely be accepted under the jurisdiction of the ME/C whereby the cause of death will be determined and whether or not there was suicidality.

In the instance where an apparent natural death has occurred at home, police investigators or ME/C investigators (also referred to as medicolegal death investigators) will seek out medical papers and prescriptions with physician or other clinical practitioner contact information and contact that individual to report the death of the patient and inquire as to whether or not he/she, if authorized, will sign the death certificate. Often, despite the natural death circumstances in a decedent with well-known and at times terminal natural disease history, the physician is reluctant to complete and sign the death certificate usually because the patient has not been seen by the physician for an extended period of time, the physician reportedly was just cross-covering the patient and is not the patient's "regular" physician, or he/she just simply does not recognize the potential of sudden death associated with many natural disease conditions. To emphasize, *any* physician who has knowledge of a patient's medical condition(s), has access to medical record information, has treated the patient, has written prescriptions for the patient, or pronounced the patient's death is eligible to certify the death. It is acknowledged that there may be uncertainty on the part of the clinician regarding the actual cause of death in a patient with natural disease who may also have a history of non-compliance with the prescribed therapeutic regimen, a psychiatric history, a history of substance use disorder, or a history of engaging in risky behavior. Such uncertainty can be resolved through consultation with ME/C officials.

There are interstate variations as to the specifics of what constitutes an ME/C case. For example, the majority or 44 of the states requires by law the investigation of suspicious or unnatural deaths and a minority or 10 of the states requires the investigation of deaths occurring within 24 hours of admission to a medical facility [3]. Local customs will also apply whereas while the law may not require the reporting or investigation of certain deaths, the practice of particular ME/C office may have always been to investigate a particular type of death and thus require its reporting.

In order for the ME/C to investigate a death, obviously, it must first be reported. Anyone, whether a layperson, police officer, or medical professional, can report a death by calling the ME/C office, any time of the day or night and all days of the year, and simply say "I would like to report a death". If the person dies outside the confines of a medical facility, whether indoors or outdoors, then the task usually falls to the police officer responding along with medical first responders to a 911 call. Once medical first responders have determined the absence of vital signs (with or without resuscitative efforts) and the medical control physician has pronounced the official date and time of the death, the police officer will report the death to the ME/C. The physician coroner or medical examiner can also pronounce the death in lieu of the medical control physician, including during physical response to certain death scenes and assume jurisdiction at that point. If the person dies in a hospital, nursing home, hospice facility, rehabilitation facility, or other medical treatment facility, then any member of the medical team including the attending physician can report the death. Not all deaths need reporting to the ME/C thus clinical practitioners must be familiar with the death reporting laws of their state. Failure to report a death that meets the criteria for reporting is a violation of state law and can result in misdemeanor-type charges. Moreover, funeral home representatives and local vital statistics officials are very knowledgeable about the types of deaths that are required to be reported to the ME/C and monitor death certificates completed by clinicians for information and circumstances that warrant reporting. In such cases, the death certificate must then be amended by the ME/C following subsequent investigation into the circumstances surrounding the death, an important fail-safe method. By that point in time however, the decedent may already have been interred or cremated hindering or precluding autopsy examination and laboratory testing of bodily fluids by the ME/C. In the unlikely event of the need to perform an autopsy for the purposes of clarifying the cause of death, disinterment of a body that has not been cremated may be necessary, an added financial and emotional hardship for the family.

3.2 What to Report and How to Report It

Often, medical facilities have a specific protocol for reporting deaths to the ME/C inclusive of categories and specific examples reflective of state regulations and local reporting customs. Contact information and instructions regarding how and what deaths to report can often be found on ME/C websites which are commonly part of government (i.e. county) online domains.

When faced with a patient that has expired in a medical facility, it must first be determined whether the circumstances that led to the death warrant reporting to the ME/C, based on state and local regulations as stated previously. Generally, if the patient expired as a result of documented or suspected injury, intoxication, or poisoning, regardless of the interval of time transpired, then the death is reportable. Under the circumstances in which a patient was hospitalized and treated at another medical facility prior to transfer to the terminal facility, the underlying reason for the presentation to the *initial* facility must be ascertained as the information may dictate whether the death ultimately is reportable. For example, a patient is admitted and treated for anoxic encephalopathy subsequent to a drug overdose and is then transferred to and dies at the second facility with an admitting diagnosis of only anoxic encephalopathy or simply “stroke”. Without ascertaining that the terminal diagnosis was as a result of the drug overdose (*or the transferring facility failed to convey the information to the receiving facility*), the death may escape reporting.

Deaths without obvious external signs of injury but that are suspected to involve abuse or neglect are reportable. This especially applies to the more vulnerable members of our society, particularly children, the elderly, and the disabled. If the circumstances surrounding the death are unknown or are suspicious, then the death is reportable. If the death is otherwise sudden and unexplained, then reporting is warranted. If one is uncertain whether or not to report a death, report it. Deaths reportable to the ME/C are found in Table 3.1:

Table 3.1 Reportable Deaths

Reportable Deaths
Deaths occurring on or after arrival to the hospital (DOA, DAA) from any cause or unknown cause
Deaths occurring within 24 hours of hospitalization (clinical definition of sudden death) except those due to chronic and/or terminal natural disease not associated with injury or toxic exposure
Deaths occurring *after* 24 hours of hospitalization and treatment without clinical explanation for the death (patients with new symptom onset, patients recovering or expected to recover from treatment, patients treated and cleared for discharge)
Deaths associated with short-term treatment and outpatient ambulatory care centers
Deaths associated with dental and oral surgery procedures
Deaths due to the acute or delayed effects of intoxicants (alcohol, illicit drugs, and medications)
Deaths due to the acute or delayed effects of injuries (craniocerebral injuries, seizures, fractures, thrombosis, sepsis, paralysis, injuries sustained during hospitalization)
Environmental deaths (extremes of temperature, natural and man-made disasters)
Maternal deaths (including trauma-associated, pregnancy-associated, abortion)
Fetal and infant deaths (including stillborns, abortions, maternal assault-related)
Sudden, unexpected or unexplained infant and child deaths
Periprocedural and therapy-associated deaths (overmedication, incorrect medication given, omission of medications, adverse effects of medications and vaccines, bedside procedure-related, surgery-related, anesthesia-related)
Work/Occupational deaths (collapsed at work, suspected toxin, radiation, or infectious disease exposure, injury-associated, chronic disease from past injury or exposure)
In-custody deaths or deaths during or following law enforcement (police) intervention
Homicidal, accidental, or suicidal injury or intoxication/poisoning (gunshot wounds, stab wounds, blunt force injury, strangulation)
Asphyxial deaths (choking/aspiration, strangulation, positional, chemical/gaseous, drowning)
Deaths associated with child or elder abuse and/or neglect
Wards of the state, institutionalized, group home residents
Deaths not attended by a physician
Unidentified or unclaimed persons

Most of the examples listed above constitute a so-called "ME's case" or "Coroner's case", in which the office would assume jurisdiction and investigate the circumstances surrounding the death inclusive of determination of cause and manner of death. However, the ME/C will not assume jurisdiction of every reported death. If the patient is well-known to a medical facility or a clinical specialist for having chronic or terminal purely natural disease (inclusive of hospice patients), where injury or intoxication are not known or suspected contributors, then the ME/C may not accept jurisdiction upon death. This is also an example of a death that does not need reporting. A death occurring at home (or otherwise outside the confines of a medical facility) under similar circumstances also does not constitute automatic acceptance of jurisdiction by the ME/C. In that case, if the treating clinician of record can be contacted and agrees to assume the responsibility for completion of the death certificate, then no jurisdiction will be assumed and this will be documented by the ME/C designated as a "report and release" case or by use of similar phraseology.

Reporting a death that has occurred in a medical facility requires communication of specific information to the **medicolegal death investigator** which is the official title that applies to a specially-trained individual certified by the **American Board of Medicolegal Death Investigators (ABMDI)**, however; not all death investigators are formally trained or boarded and otherwise may have equivalent experience in death investigation and perform all of the requisite functions. The reporting agency (hospital, outpatient treatment facility, nursing home, rehabilitation facility, assisted living facility, or other medical facility) should be prepared to convey the following information:

- Reporter name, title, and location
- Decedent's full legal name, home address, phone number
- Decedent's date of birth, age, race , sex
- Decedent's social security number
- Decedent's marital status, spouse name, contact information
- Name of legal next-of-kin or family member/representative and contact information (see Appendix A)
- Means of arrival to medical facility (car, EMS, etc.)
- Date and time of arrival to facility
- Brief history and circumstances and medical history
- Synopsis of clinical findings
- Synopsis of therapeutic intervention(s)
- Date and time of pronouncement of death
- Pronouncing physician's name

The decedent's identity may be uncertain or unknown and special efforts by the ME/C's office to establish or confirm identity will commence if/once jurisdiction is accepted. Additionally, it is especially important to convey historical or clinical evidence of injury or intoxication/poisoning **regardless of the interval**

of time between the injury or intoxication/poisoning and death. Delayed deaths stemming from an injury or intoxication/poisoning can occur days, weeks, months, and even years after the initial event as a result of complications like bacterial pneumonia, pulmonary thromboembolism, urosepsis, and even hypertensive stroke in spinal cord injury patients with autonomic dysreflexia. Moreover, pre-existing chronic natural disease like hypertensive cardiovascular disease and chronic lung disease can also be exacerbated by the pathophysiological effects of acute injury whereupon the patient never returned to baseline function, and therefore a connection exists. Particularly in the elderly, fractures of the vertebrae, ribs, hip, pelvis and long bones of the upper and lower extremities, are likely contributors to death, when the death occurs within one year of sustaining the fracture [4]. Acute pain, immobility, and debility resulting from injury cause physiologic stress, including that mediated by catecholamines, on compromised organ systems that have limited functional reserve. Thus, deaths occurring within one year of sustaining a fracture or during *any* time frame where the patient did not return to baseline function and/or developed complications and decompensated further should be reported.

There are a number of other medical diagnoses and non-specific conditions that can be a complication of natural disease, injury (including iatrogenic), intoxication/poisoning, self-neglect or inflicted physical abuse and neglect. Some of the conditions may recur or persist for days, weeks, months, and years prior to death and often become part of the list of primary medical diagnoses with omission of the specific etiology. Importantly, delayed deaths arising from complications of neglect, abuse, injury or poisoning caused by another individual(s) are homicidal in nature. Therefore, clinicians treating certain conditions with potentially non-natural causes must not lose sight of the specific underlying etiology or etiologies as they become known as this will not only preclude the formulation of the most accurate cause-of-death statement but also result in a failure to report the death to the ME/C, should the patient expire. A few of the more prominent examples are listed in Table 3.2:

Table 3.2 Selection of diagnoses and conditions with possible non-natural causes

Central and Peripheral Nervous Systems • Cerebral edema • Cerebral herniation • Cerebral infarction • Encephalopathy -hypoxic/anoxic -hypoxic/ischemic -metabolic • Epilepsy, seizures • Hemorrhage -intracranial -epidural -subdural -subarachnoid • Mental status alteration • Paralysis -paraplegia -quadriplegia	Cardiovascular System • Acute myocardial infarct • Aortic avulsion, tear • Aortic dissection or aneurysm • Arrhythmia • Bacterial endocarditis • Cardiac arrest • Cardiac tamponade • Cardiogenic shock • Hemopericardium • Ischemia • Myocardial rupture	Respiratory System • Anoxia/hypoxia • Asphyxia • Atelectasis • Empyema • Hemothorax • Laryngeal edema • Pleural effusion • Pneumonia • Pneumothorax • Pulmonary edema • Pulmonary embolism (blood clot, air, fat) • Respiratory failure
Gastrointestinal System • Adhesions, visceral • Bowel/intestinal ischemia or infarction • Bowel/intestinal strangulation , incarceration, or obstruction • Hemorrhage • Perforated bowel or viscus • Peritonitis	Multisystem, system non-specific • Anemia • Bed-bound • Debility • Dehydration • Exsanguination • Failure-to-thrive • Hypo/hyperthermia • Infections, recurrent (i.e. urinary tract infection with urosepsis) • Malnutrition • Metabolic acidosis • Multiple system organ failure • Overdose (medications, illicit drugs, ethanol) • Rhabdomyolysis • Sepsis • Systemic Inflammatory Response Syndrome	Musculoskeletal/soft tissue • Burns (thermal, chemical) • Cellulitis, fasciitis • Compartment syndrome • Contractures • Decubital ulcers • Fat embolism • Fat necrosis • Fractures • Gangrene • Hematoma • Muscle atrophy • Osteomyelitis • Subcutaneous emphysema • Thrombophlebitis • Venous thrombosis • Wounds

Certain conditions like failure-to-thrive, dehydration, malnutrition, and debility are more commonly the result of natural disease sequela or the aging process but may also be the consequence of abuse and neglect. Paralysis can be the result of natural conditions such as multiple sclerosis as well as traumatic spinal cord and brain injury. Anoxia and hypoxia are conditions that can arise as a result of the acute or delayed effects of asphyxia caused by drowning, narcotic overdose, and choking. Penetrating injury can result in air or blood accumulation within body cavities or within soft tissues. Blood-loss anemia may be associated with acute injury or represent complication following injury including iatrogenic types. Arterial dissection, arterial tears, and scar tissue within body cavities may represent acute or remote blunt force or penetrating trauma. Fractures are less commonly pathologic thus blunt force trauma must be the primary etiologic consideration. While acute myocardial infarction more commonly is the result of coronary artery disease, it may also develop following hypotension caused by a drug overdose or develop as part of trauma-associated hemorrhage. Deep vein thrombosis causing fatal thromboembolic events may be due not only to hypercoagulable states conferred by natural disease entities by also occur as a result of immobility caused by injury or traumatic vascular injury of the upper and lower extremities. Certain poisons and other intoxicants can cause acid-base disturbances. Adverse medication or drug reactions may cause alterations in blood counts, present with electrocardiographic abnormalities, or manifest as hyperthermia. Wounds with or without underlying soft tissue infection and decubital ulcers may represent inflicted injury, accidental injury or the long term complication of debilitating injury.

If it is known that the decedent in fact sustained injury, intoxication, or some type of neglect or abuse that led to one or more of medical diagnoses or conditions listed in the preceding table and they are listed on the death certificate without reference to what caused them, then the manner of death cannot be certified as natural, as is often found on erroneous death certificates. **When it cannot be determined whether or not certain diagnoses or conditions were caused by injury, intoxication, neglect, or abuse, then the death must be reported in lieu of signing the death certificate**. The inclusion of these non-specific entities on a death certificate will trigger a query process (see Chapter 8, section 8.1) targeting the certifier of the death or cause it to be referred to the local ME/C for further investigation. If referred to the ME/C, an investigation into the circumstances surrounding the death via obtaining the relevant history, reviewing pertinent records including medical records, and requesting police investigation if warranted, will be done. Performance of an autopsy may also be necessary to clarify the cause of death if the decedent has not already been buried or cremated. If an autopsy is necessary and the decedent has already been buried, disinterment will be necessary at additional expense (and distress) to the family. Furthermore, *time will be of the essence if circumstances suggestive of foul play or homicidal violence are discovered as a period of time has already transpired with the initial death certification process and that transpired time may equate to loss of vital evidence and access to witnesses*. Subsequent to review of all information and any autopsy results, a revised cause-of-death statement along with selection of the appropriate manner of death will be entered on an amended death certificate and then re-registered.

Upon logging in of all reported information, a determination will be made as to whether or not the circumstances constitute an ME/C case in accordance with state and local regulations and local customs, and if so, jurisdiction will be accepted and arrangements will be made for transportation of the decedent along with the personal effects to the ME/C's office. An on-call forensic pathologist may be contacted by the investigator for advice on deaths with equivocal circumstances, in offices fortunate enough to have them. Otherwise, such decision-making responsibilities fall to the Medical Examiner or Coroner in charge of the office or his/her deputy.

Families or legal representatives should then be informed that the ME/C has accepted jurisdiction, will take possession of the personal effects and the body, and ultimately will determine the cause and manner of death with completion of the death certificate. **They should also be informed that an autopsy may or may not be necessary**. It is often assumed by families and medical personnel alike that an autopsy will automatically be performed on every ME/C case. The decision to perform an autopsy is made on a case-by-case basis after first reviewing the history and circumstances. Approximately 25% to 50% of ME/C cases are autopsied and the range is a reflection of interoffice variability regarding local practice, funding, and staffing. Families or persons representing the decedent may have requested that an autopsy be performed. **The request for an autopsy by the family or representative must be conveyed to the ME/C's office at the time the death is reported and recorded in the medical record**. Families or decedent representatives may also express a religious objection to an autopsy and request that no autopsy be performed, or for other reasons request that one not be performed. **The request that no autopsy be performed must also**

be specifically conveyed at the time the death is reported to the ME/C and recorded in the medical record. Between the time after the death has been reported and accepted by the ME/C, families or decedent representatives, having obtained contact information for the ME/C's office, may at times contact that office directly to express wishes for or against performance of an autopsy. The treating physicians at times may also request that an autopsy be performed on decedent's that have come under the jurisdiction of the ME/C which will be determined on a case-by-case basis and with consideration of any known family concerns and objections.

As a component of standard operating procedure for a death occurring at a medical facility, the "Report to the Medical Examiner/Coroner Form" summarizing the decedent's terminal encounter, decedent identifying information, and the clinician's opinion of the cause of death must be completed with a copy to accompany the body or be promptly sent electronically to the ME/C (see sample Report to the ME/C Form Appendix B). This documentation becomes part of the medical record. An additional component to the documentation of a hospital death entails completion of a death report which records identifying decedent information, legal next-of-kin contact information, ME/C's jurisdiction, request for autopsy by legal next-of-kin, release of decedent and decedent property information, and certifying physician information (see sample Death Report and Release Form Appendix C). A copy of this form must also accompany the body or be forwarded to the ME/C and otherwise becomes part of decedent's medical record.

If jurisdiction is declined by the ME/C, explanation will be provided with documentation of the same. A quality assurance measure by way of ongoing review and verification of so-called "report and release cases", which may go by similar phraseology at any given office, is a standard practice of accredited ME/C offices. As an added quality assurance measure, the investigator will inquire and document specifically the name and contact information of the individual who will complete the death certificate and the most likely cause of death that will be listed. **The physician (most commonly the attending physician) or other duly authorized or designated medical professional is responsible for the completion of the death certificate for deaths in which the ME/C has declined jurisdiction.** The reporting facility is responsible for after-death care and preparation of the decedent and assisting families or legal representatives with making contact with the funeral home that will retrieve the decedent from the medical facility, tasks handled specifically by the morgue attendant.

The sudden and unexpected death of an infant is a special category of death in which key specific questions regarding the terminal circumstances and the infant's overall health will be asked by the medicolegal death investigator. The investigator may also physically respond to the medical facility to view the infant and obtain the same information. This is in accordance to the information required of the Sudden Unexplained Infant Death Investigation Reporting Form (SUIDI-RF) as part of the CDC's Sudden Unexplained Infant Death initiative, an effort to better define environmental risk factors and medical/birth history associated with these deaths by standardizing and improving data collection [5]. Much of the information on the SUIDI-RF form is obtained from the caretakers and includes a home visit with doll re-enactment and scene recreation by the death investigator in order to get detailed information of events leading up to the unresponsiveness or death. Of great importance is the "Summary for Pathologist" section which provides a synopsis of the death circumstances and flags findings such as unsafe or change in sleep environment, recent injuries, and undiagnosed medical conditions. The infant may also be conveyed to the hospital having undergone resuscitative efforts and received a clinical examination and workup during which time the examiners may note signs of illness or atypical injury. Review of the clinical information generated on and after arrival to the hospital is also an essential part of the workup of infant deaths.

Normally, the privacy rules of the **Health Insurance Portability and Accountability Act (HIPAA)** protect patients' health information throughout the normal course of care. There are important exceptions to the rules and the exceptions permit disclosure of medical information relevant to a death investigation commenced by the ME/C, law enforcement investigation into criminal matters involving a living or deceased individual, or investigation regarding abuse and neglect of a *living or deceased* individual [6]. The author has had past personal experience in which hospital personnel, unfamiliar with the HIPAA exceptions, have refused to provide medical information and death circumstances to homicide detectives investigating infant deaths, instead referring them to the hospital's risk management office. This can be highly problematic as any information relative to an infant or child death is vital to the forensic pathologist who will be performing the autopsy and to the detectives attempting to investigate allegations of abuse and neglect. In accordance to the

HIPAA exemptions, not only will medical information be requested verbally at the time the death is reported, but also subsequent to acceptance of jurisdiction. Importantly, medical records will be requested at some time during the death investigation, including but not limited to the following:

- Emergency department records
- Admission history and physical examination records
- Progress and nurses notes (especially within 24 hours of death)
- Injury/incident reports
- Laboratory, operative, and radiology reports
- Discharge and expiration summaries

To summarize, when reporting your patient's death to the ME/C, it is essential to know the laws and regulations regarding death reporting and to be prepared to convey key pieces of historical and clinical information so that the proper jurisdictional decision can be made. The fully completed official report to the ME/C (see Appendix B sample form), containing identifying patient information and summarizing the terminal clinical events, is an important preliminary source of information and additional medical records will likely be requested. The acceptance of jurisdiction over a death reported by a medical facility is at the discretion of the ME/C based on the history, circumstances, and the laws, and the ME/C is not obligated to accept jurisdiction over all reported deaths. Finally, **it is the responsibility of the physician or authorized designee to promptly complete the death certificate on all deaths in which the ME/C has declined jurisdiction**. Appendix D provides concise flowcharts of the essential tasks for reporting a death.

References

1. Ohio Revised Code, Title 3-Counties, Chapter 313. Available at: www.codes.ohio.gov. Accessed 1/10/2016.

2. Hickman MJ, Hughes KA, Strom KJ, and Ropero-Miller JD. Medical Examiners' and Coroners' Offices, 2004. Available at: www.bjs.gov/content/pub/pdf/meco04.pdf. Accessed 12/29/2015.

3. Caucci L and Warner M. Selected characteristics of death requiring investigation by state-table 1. Available at: www.cdc.gov/phlp/publications/coroner/investigations.html. Accessed 12/15/2015.

4. Dolinak, D. Review of the significance of various low force fractures in the elderly. *Am J Forensic Med Pathol.* 2008;29(2):99-105.

5. Sudden Unexplained Infant Death Investigation Reporting Form (SUIDI-RF). Available at: www.cdc.gov/sids/suidrf.htm. Accessed 12/30/2015.

6. Health Information Privacy. US Department of Health and Human Services. Available at: www.hhs.gov/ocr/privacy. Accessed 12/12/2015.

CHAPTER 4

MEDICAL EXAMINER-CORONER CASES AT MEDICAL FACILITIES

4.1 Decedent Handling

Having had an official date and time of pronouncement of death, the once patient becomes the **decedent**. Note the contrast in spelling and definition of the often incorrectly substituted term-*descendant*. Following this, notification of family members or representatives is in order. Particularly, it is important to convey to the family or representatives that by virtue of the death circumstances, the Medical Examiner or Coroner (ME/C) has taken jurisdiction over the death and will further investigate and determine the official cause of death.

The mortician, morgue attendant, or other designated personnel of the medical facility will provide postmortem care such as taping the eyes closed to protect from drying, placing arms in a neutral position and closing the mouth before onset of rigor mortis, and placing a clean sheet over the body. The properly identified and tagged decedent will then be placed temporarily into the facility's refrigerated morgue. Ultimately, a transport service will be dispatched to the medical facility and transport workers will place the decedent into a clean body bag that is then sealed with subsequent transport to the ME/C's office. The mortician or other designated individual may also be charged with executing the completion of the Death Report and Release Form (see Appendix C). It is important that an open line of communication is initiated and maintained between the mortician and the clinical team regarding coordination of end-of-life preparations for decedents destined for the ME/C's office. In other facilities, a patient liaison, social worker or member of the decedent's clinical team may fulfill the role of the mortician preferably according to established protocol specifically for the handling of decedents that have come under the jurisdiction of the ME/C.

Even before treatment and resuscitative efforts have been ended, there are some important tasks that the patient's clinical team must ensure are done. These tasks relate to the circumstances surrounding the death and to the collection and preservation of clothing, personal effects, and foreign materials that may be present with, on, or within the decedent. This is applicable particularly to homicidal or suspicious circumstances whether the decedent is the alleged victim or suspect. This is also applicable to deaths occurring while in police custody or during or following police intervention.

4.1.1 Therapeutic Devices

Foremost, **all therapeutic devices placed on or in the patient must be left in place**. This includes all indwelling tubes for intubation and gastric or fecal drainage, surgical drains, chest tubes, intravascular and intraosseous catheters, pulse oximeter sensors, cervical collars, bandages, casts and electrocardiogram/defibrillation pads. This facilitates the differentiation of therapy-associated injury from other types of injury including inflicted injury. It also allows for assessment of proper placement of catheters and tubes and for the identification of perforation and intravascular thrombosis caused by intravascular catheters. As examples, chest tube incisions can appear like stab wounds, venipunctures can mimic the stigmata associated with intravenous drug abuse, and defibrillation pads can leave burn-like injuries. Scalp-vein catheterization or placement of scalp monitors on infants can leave ecchymotic areas or subgaleal hemorrhages that look like impact sites. Hemo/pneumothorax may complicate central line and chest tube placement. Therapeutic devices will be later documented upon external-only examination or examination during autopsy and the medical records will be reviewed for correlation if necessary. If a patient with penetrating or perforating injuries (i.e. gunshot wounds, stab wounds, and lacerations) arrives and is pronounced dead on arrival or very soon after arrival to the hospital, cleaning or suturing of wounds should be avoided as this may remove or distort valuable evidence such as gunpowder residue or metal and paint fragments originating from a bullet, knife, or blunt object. Instead, the securement of multilayered gauze bandaging over the wound is preferred. If at all possible, excluding the necessity of life-saving measures, **the use of penetrating or perforating wounds as access ports for catheters should be avoided** as this can modify or obliterate certain characteristics of wounds that help to identify them. Certain surgical or other life-saving wound modifications such as the use of sponge-filled syringes may be necessary to mitigate hemorrhaging from wounds, however.

4.1.2 Medicolegal Evidence

Medicolegal evidence comes in many different forms including clothing, bullets, hairs, fibers, blood, and particulate matter, both seen and unseen. The decedent's body is also a receptacle of medicolegal evidence, from the types and distribution of injuries to the type of foreign material residing upon or within. More precisely, **trace evidence** is what is left behind when one object or surface contacts another, as defined by Locard's Exchange Principle, named after the early 20th century forensic science pioneer. In forensic work, collection and preservation of evidence in its original state is of utmost importance. It further involves starting and maintaining what is called the **chain of custody** which is a tracking system that documents the physical location and status of analysis of a collected item or piece of evidence and the persons involved in the handling of the same. As the decedent's body may harbor evidence, it is standard protocol for the body to be placed into a clean, zippered body bag to which identification tags or barcodes are attached and documented prior transport to the ME/C's office by a designated transportation/courier service.

Medicolegal evidence may be examined, tested and later presented by forensic experts in a court of law affecting decisions by judge and jury regarding a defendant's guilt or innocence, freedom or imprisonment. For this reason, foreign materials, clothing, currency, medications, drugs and drug paraphernalia, cell phones and other items must be properly collected accordingly, preferably separately in paper bags, and put in a designated secure location prior to submission to a ME/C representative or law enforcement official. The use of *paper* receptacles (as opposed to plastic) is essential as paper does not promote mold and bacterial growth that could interfere with scientific forensic analysis such as DNA testing. If articles of clothing have not been previously removed by medical first responders and removal is necessary, they should be cut along the seams avoiding pre-existing tears or other defects which may correspond to wounds made by bullets, knife blades or other penetrating objects or otherwise that may have imbedded foreign material. Attempts to wash, wipe or clean personal effects must be avoided. Table 4.1 lists the essential tasks and rationale regarding handling of evidence. In sexual assault cases, where the death may have been pronounced after a period of hospitalization, a forensic nurse may have performed relevant collections and would proceed with further submission according to the established chain-of-custody protocols.

4.1.3 Weapons and Ammunition

Weapons like firearms and knives may be stuck in or fall out of clothing or be inside of pockets or waistbands. Police must be notified immediately if any weapons or ammunition are found. Weapons constitute evidence which must be handled and collected properly according to the established policy of the medical facility.

Firearms must not be cleaned by medical personnel and should be handled as little as is necessary to remove it from the treatment field taking care not to point the muzzle end at anyone, depress the trigger or separate the weapon from its holster if inside of one. It will be necessary for a law enforcement official to ensure that the firearm is "safe" and free of ammunition and cannot otherwise be discharged with the potential of causing harm to others. Bullets or bullet fragments, which may also be adhered to or fall out of clothing, must be handled with clean gloved hands and not handled with metal implements like forceps as this could leave markings that interfere with later examination by a ballistics examiner. Any soft tissue, fabric, or other foreign material adherent to bullets must be left in place as these have evidentiary value. Bullets or related metallic fragments that fall out of wounds during treatment or are recovered during surgery must be similarly handled and placed in secured receptacles labeled with patient identifiers and the date, stored in a designated secure location, and transferred to law enforcement of ME/C officials according to chain-of-custody protocol. If bullets or bullet fragments are observed within the depths of wounds of the decedent, care must be taken to ensure that they do not fall out by securing gauze wrappings or broad bandages over the wounds and alerting law enforcement and ME/C officials. Deformed or fragmented bullets can be sharp and thus universal precautions must be exercised when handled.

TASER® devices (TASER International www.taser.com) are hand-held conducted electrical devices used by law enforcement to subdue and elicit compliance. They can also be legally owned and used by private citizens for self-defense. These devices fire 2 dart-like electrodes at a distance of up to 35 feet and further activation produces pain and involuntary muscle contraction upon contact with clothing and skin. Uncommonly, deaths have resulted in association with and following use of the devices and therefore subsequent medical evaluation of individuals who have sustained shocks from these devices is warranted or otherwise prompted by a sudden change in responsiveness, causing law enforcement to summon medical first responders, particularly in police-involved incidents. It may also become necessary to convey these individuals to the hospital for further resuscitation and treatment. The metallic, dart-like electrodes are barbed and remain imbedded within clothing and skin and thus may be encountered by medical first responders and hospital personnel. If the darts remain embedded in skin, medical first responders and hospital personnel should document the anatomic location of the darts in the medical record including photographically if possible. Removal should be done only by trained law enforcement and medical personnel manually or with the assistance of a special extractor tool. Care must also be exercised to securely preserve the darts that have become embedded in clothing by removal or by preservation of the clothing upon which the darts are embedded, with the appropriate documentation in the medical record and alerting of law enforcement prior to release of the articles. Any removed darts must be properly contained, preferably in a rigid sealable container or containers provided with the extractor tool kit. They are considered as sharp biohazardous implements much like hypodermic needles and universal precautions must be exercised upon handling. They also represent evidence and must be inventoried and stored in a designated secured location.

Handling of knives by the handle should be avoided so as not to disrupt markings like fingerprints or DNA-containing biological material like blood. If a knife or similar implement remains in the decedent with the handle protruding, then a paper bag must be secured over the handle. If it is otherwise separate from the body it should be handled with clean gloved hands by the area not normally handled such as the non-sharp part of the instrument between the blade and the handle known as the hilt or ricasso. The instrument must then be placed in a rigid marked/labeled receptacle such as a cardboard box and stored in a secured location prior to transfer to law enforcement.

Pieces, parts, or various coatings from blunt objects like wooden boards, tools, and other yieldable weapons may also become embedded in clothing or in wounds as a result of impact(s). Care should be exercised to not disturb fragmented materials and ensure that they are contained and secured with the clothing. Any materials adherent to or embedded within wounds must be secured with bandaging.

4.1.4 Drug Paraphernalia and Medications

Illicit drugs and paraphernalia may accompany the decedent and be found on or in clothing, amongst or within personal effects, or within body cavities or orifices. This includes small plastic baggies containing drugs or powdery residues, blunts, glass pipes, syringes, steel wool, spoons, straws, and rolled up paper currency. Caution must be exercised when reaching into pockets or purses and wallets which may contain uncapped syringes or broken glass pipes. Increasingly potent illicit drugs, diverted medications, and related analogues like heroin, fentanyl and carfentanil, have the potential to cause intoxication at very small doses. For that reason, gloves must be worn when handling drug paraphernalia or clothing and should be changed prior to touching other objects or examining patients to safeguard against the transfer of residues unknowingly. Masks can also safeguard against inhalational exposure. Loose or mislabeled tablets misused by ingestion, crushing with snorting, or by dissolving with injection, may also be found. Patients may also clandestinely acquire illicit drugs and associated paraphernalia while hospitalized. Analgesic transdermal medication patches may be misused by placing them into the mouth or by extraction of the contents directly from the patches with subsequent injection, either of which can lead to death by overdose. Patients may also ingest small plastic baggies containing illicit drugs in order to escape detection by police prior to apprehension or to escape detection by hospital personnel upon suspicion of possession and risk death by overdose. Any recovered drugs, drug paraphernalia, or non-administered medications must not be discarded but instead be placed in a designated secure location and notification of the ME/C and police must promptly follow. Scientific identification and documentation of these items may be pertinent to the death circumstances, cause-of-death determination, and to ongoing or subsequent police investigation.

4.1.5 Chain of Custody and Evidence Handling

It is protocol in many medical facilities to perform an inventory of personal effects and other items of evidentiary value using a special chain of custody form for documentation which becomes part of the permanent medical record. Importantly, the printed name and signature of the person that performs the inventory of the items in addition to the printed name and signature of the ME/C representative or law enforcement officer who receives any items must be entered onto the form (see sample Chain of Custody Form in Appendix E). The chain-of-custody/inventory record is essential as it is used as a tracking mechanism for evidence and may later be presented in court. Protocols for handling medicolegal evidence recovered during surgery or during surgical pathology examination inclusive of chain-of-custody specifics are practiced according to institutional policy [1]. Furthermore, protocols for large-scale events such mass casualties have been proposed in the literature [2]. Law enforcement and/or ME/C officials should be notified of any foreign materials collected from the body for subsequent retrieval. The personal effects from an individual *not* known or suspected to have died while in custody or under homicidal or suspicious circumstances may be handled according to the usual protocol of the medical facility and submitted along with the body to be conveyed to the ME/C's office. As a routine and standard, clothing and personal effects belonging to a decedent destined for the ME/C's office will stay with the decedent and later be released from the ME/C's office to the funeral home after verification that the circumstances surrounding the death do not warrant retention and further forensic examination.

4.1.6 Interaction with Law Enforcement

Law enforcement officials including police officers and detectives may already be aware of the homicidal or suspicious circumstances and have caused paper bags to be placed on the hands and sometimes the feet at the death scene or shortly after arrival to the hospital, in order to contain any adherent trace evidence. The bags must not be removed unless life-saving therapeutic measures are necessary. Collection of trace evidence from the hands may also be performed by law enforcement officials at the hospital as well. Law enforcement officials will inquire about other items like weapons, clothing, cellphones and other personal effects that accompany the decedent and any other foreign material recovered from the decedent during treatment. They will collect these items according to chain-of-custody protocol along with documentation of the same on an evidence log. **Under no circumstances should personal effects and weapons be given to family members, family representatives, or acquaintances, particularly if the death is homicidal or suspicious or involves police custody.** These individuals also must not be permitted to have physical contact with a decedent in which the death circumstances are suspicious for foul play in order to prevent the unintentional or deliberate contamination or alteration of any on-body evidence. This may be difficult upon arrival of grieving family members who may express emotions of anger and extreme distress. Involvement of in-house security personnel and any law enforcement personnel already in attendance may be necessary to ensure that the no-contact policy is enforced.

4.2 Biological Sample/Specimen Retention

In light of the history of present illness, clinical presentation and clinical course, concerns that a death may have resulted from an illicit drug or medication overdose or poisoning by some other substance may arise. That information will or should have already been conveyed upon reporting of the death and the medicolegal death investigator will request that a hold to be placed on admission blood and urine samples or other types of bodily fluids like meconium or umbilical cord blood in newborn infant deaths. These samples will be retrieved from the medical facility by a ME/C representative, or a request to send samples by mail or courier service to the ME/C's office will be done if geographical distance is an issue.

Admission blood samples stored in the chemistry laboratory or the pre-transfusion blood samples stored in the blood bank laboratory are particularly advantageous for the ME/C to obtain and test. The earliest blood samples drawn shortly after admission or during the first few hours of admission are best because they would contain the highest level of any potential intoxicant and/or its metabolites prior to any reduction in concentration owing to dilution by intravenous fluids given for resuscitation or the body's own metabolism and elimination. The earliest blood sample is also important because some drugs like heroin have very short half-lives and are metabolized rapidly. Other drugs like certain fentanyl analogues may be present at very low blood concentrations on admission and rapidly become undetectable during the hospital course.

Hospital blood samples are generally not retained for long periods of time, often only from 3 to 7 days and the window of opportunity to obtain these important samples may have already closed in the case of a prolonged hospital course. If it has been determined that patient's medical condition is critical or that death is imminent and an overdose or poisoning is suspected, then proactive measures to retain any admission blood, pre-transfusion blood, and urine samples should be done as soon as possible in anticipation of postmortem testing which can greatly aid in the determination of the cause of death. Postmortem testing of blood samples drawn within the first few hours or days after admission can also reveal the presence of intoxicants and their metabolites and these specimens may also be requested. Blood samples drawn into tubes containing anticoagulant (EDTA) and sodium fluoride preservative are preferred but any remaining blood specimens including blood drawn into serum separator or red/red-gray tubes can be useful. While the emphasis has been on obtaining blood samples, *urine* samples will also be sought as testing of urine can reveal evidence of acute and/or historic intake of a substance relevant to the medical history, clinical presentation and clinical course. Samples from deaths in which overdose is suspected will be qualitatively and quantitatively analyzed in the forensic toxicology laboratory.

Concerns for inadvertent overmedication, omission of medication, or adverse reaction to medications given during hospitalization may arise as suggested by the clinical course, new symptom onset, and the history and circumstances leading to hospitalization and death. Families may also raise these same concerns particularly in a loved one who seemed to have been making a recovery prior to a rapid decline and death. If these concerns are reported to the ME/C, multiple samples, especially blood samples drawn over the time of hospitalization may be requested.

Other types of biological specimens like pre-transfusion blood samples stored in the blood bank or tissue specimens stored in the clinical or surgical pathology laboratories may be requested as these specimens are a source of DNA which may be needed for the purposes of establishing or confirming the identity in an unidentified or tentatively identified individual. Whole or remnant placental or fetal tissues that may be retained in the surgical pathology laboratory or obstetrical departments may be requested as they too represent a source of DNA that can be used to help establish or confirm parentage.

Craniectomy and other surgically removed osseous specimens with perforations caused by bullets and sharp instruments or that have fractures caused by blunt objects are routinely retained in the laboratories of operating rooms as they may be re-attached to the surviving patient at a later time as clinically indicated. Osseous tissue not suitable for re-attachment may be submitted to the surgical pathology laboratory where they will be handled and retained according to standard procedure. Documentation of the characteristics and patterns of injury imparted by the bullet or other object and collection with submission of any foreign material that may be imbedded are essential tasks that the forensic pathologist must perform. Subsequent interpretation of osseous injury and analysis of any collected trace evidence are critical for cause and manner of death determination and reconstruction of the death circumstances, especially in homicidal deaths. These specimens will be requested at the direction of or directly by the forensic pathologist conducting the autopsy.

4.3 Tissue and Organ Procurement Issues

The need for tissues and organs remains great across the United States with the number of lives saved and the thousands of patients that still die while waiting for an organ transplant notable [3]. Statutes exist that permit tissue procurement organizations (TPOs) to approach the next-of-kin to request an anatomical gift of an organ or tissue from an eligible decedent and obtain consent for harvesting after neurological or cardiac death. Permission for procurement may have already been self-predetermined and appear on a state registry or driver's license. If the decedent did not previously consent to organ harvesting, consent must be obtained from the next-of-kin. A detailed medical and social history will be obtained from the medical records and the consentee to help identify risk factors for malignancy and communicable disease and determine suitability for donation. This information is made available to the ME/C as well. Procurement of tissues and organs, especially solid organs, may take place at the medical facility, while the decedent remains on mechanical life supports and after determination of neurological or cardiac death. Procurement of tissues like skin, bones, eyes for corneas, and heart for valves, may take place at the ME/C's office within 24 hours after the death.

The ME/C is charged with the determination of cause and manner of death which involves review of the historical information and external examination of the body at the very least, and sometimes the performance of an autopsy. The ME/C also recognizes the importance and benefit of tissue and organ procurement and transplantation. In deaths occurring under suspicious or homicidal circumstances, the ME/C must balance the absolute necessity of collection and preservation of evidence and the determination of cause and manner of death with wishes of the families to provide an anatomical gift, the needs of the tissue procurement organizations (TPOs), and the waiting recipients that stand to benefit. The National Association of Medical Examiners' position on the release of organs and tissues states that this can be done in the vast majority of cases without compromise of the legal duty of the ME/C [4]. However, in certain cases, it may be necessary for the ME/C to restrict the procurement of certain tissues and/or organs that could compromise cause and manner of death determination, particularly in decedents with no medical history and sudden deaths in infants and children.

ME/Cs and TPOs across the country have established cooperative working relationships and protocols whereby after obtainment of consent, the harvesting of tissues and organs can proceed in a manner that does not interfere with collection of evidence or determination of cause and manner of death by the forensic scientist and forensic pathologist, respectively. Examples include procurement of tissue and organs after trace evidence collection have been performed but prior to autopsy performance, procurement after performance of an external examination of the body not slated for autopsy performance or procurement after both an external examination and an autopsy has been performed. Procurement may even take place *prior* to trace evidence collection after bagging of the hands by the procurement technicians. TPO technicians may consult with a ME/C pathologist on unusual findings encountered during procurement or will otherwise abort the procurement procedure altogether if unusual or unexpected injury or signs of infectious or neoplastic disease are found. Surgeons assisting TPOs with solid organ procurement may also request an intraoperative consultation with a ME/C pathologist or abort the procurement procedure altogether for the same reasons. Furthermore, the concern of missing a cardiac cause of death in a decedent who has had harvesting of the heart for valves is ameliorated by the routine examination by a cardiac pathologist of the organ after removal of the valves followed by issuance of a gross and microscopic report, return of microscopic slides, and return of residual wet tissue if requested.

As part of the cooperative working relationship between TPOs and ME/Cs, peripheral blood samples (i.e. subclavian blood) and vitreous fluid can be easily obtained in properly labeled specimen containers and provided to the ME/C. These specimens may be later tested for the presence of intoxicants or medications. Technicians will also provide documentation of external and internal findings of the body prior to and during procurement such as therapeutic devices and injuries. Additionally, the types of tissue or organs recovered will be documented inclusive of notation on a tag attached to an extremity. Any attachments on the body containing procurement information should be left in place as this information will be reviewed in conjunction with examination of the body at the ME/C's office.

Table 4.1 Essentials of Medicolegal Evidence Handling

Action	Reason
Wear clean disposable gloves when handling evidence	Reduces/prevents handler contamination of evidence
Avoid cutting through clothing defects	Alters or destroys evidence
Never clean, wash or wipe off clothing or personal effects	Alters or destroys evidence
Use appropriately sized and sealable containers for surgical specimens	Assures secure containment
Never handle guns	May be loaded with ammunition, may cause discharge and bystander injury
Never handle bullets with metal implements	Causes extraneous markings that interfere with ballistics examination
Use paper bags to secure over handles of indwelling sharp instruments like knives	Preserves evidence on handle
Place personal effects and clothing in paper bags, not plastic	Retards/prevents growth of microorganisms that can destroy DNA
Clearly label all containers and receptacles with patient/decedent identifiers, date, and contents	Essential part of the chain-of-custody procedure
Never discard clothing or personal effects regardless of condition	To prevent loss of evidence and impedance of investigation
Never give personal effects to family members, representatives, or acquaintances	To prevent loss of evidence and impedance of investigation
Enforce no-contact policy with decedent	To prevent loss of evidence and impedance of investigation
Maintain an inventory record of all items	Important for point of reference for law enforcement official or ME/C
Store decedent personal effects and recovered materials in secured, monitored location	Ensures integrity of items and materials, assures unbroken chain-of-custody

References

1. Association of Surgical Technologists Standards for Handling and Care of Surgical Specimens, Section XI. Available at: www.ast.org/uploadfiles/Main_Site_/Content/About_Us/Standard_Handling_Care_Surgical_Specimen.pdf. Accessed 1/1/2016.

2. Byrne-Dugan CJ, Cederroth TA, Deshpande A, and Remick DG. The processing of surgical specimens with forensic evidence: Lessons learned from the Boston Marathon bombings. *Arch Pathol Lab Med.* 2015;139:1024-1027.

3. Organ Procurement and Transplantation Network. US Department of Health and Human Services. Available at: https://optn.transplant.hrsa.gov/. Accessed 1/31/2016.

4. Pinckard JK, Wetli CV, Graham MA. National Association of Medical Examiners position paper on the medical examiner release of organs and tissues for transplantation. *Am J Forensic Med Pathol.* 2007;28(3):202-207.

CHAPTER 5

HOSPITAL versus FORENSIC AUTOPSIES

Introduction

Autopsy-the term derived from the Greek word *autopsia* means to see with one's own eyes. It is a medical procedure that involves the detailed gross examination of organs, tissues, and fluids and it is the gold standard in the practice of forensic pathology for the determination of the cause of death. The autopsy can reveal previously unknown, undiagnosed, and misdiagnosed medical conditions and is an important quality assurance tool for clinical medical practice and for the reduction and prevention of medical error-associated death [1,2,3,4]. Countless articles published by pathologists in general pathology, forensic medicine and pathology, and clinical medicine journals alike are a testament to these facts. Surveillance and diagnosis of emerging and re-emerging infectious disease and documentation of the evolution and extent of chronic disease have been and continues to be greatly aided by the autopsy. It can also confirm proper surgical procedure or reveal acute and delayed surgical complications inclusive of surgeries involving implantation of organs, tissues, and prostheses. In the clinical setting, the hospital autopsy is an invaluable tool for clinicopathologic correlation and a teaching tool for doctors and doctors-in-training. **It is instrumental in providing clinicians with the etiologically specific cause-of-death, information that is necessary for completion of the death certificate.** Not only is it required, it is also vitally essential that the pathology resident master the techniques of the hospital autopsy (synonymous with clinical or medical autopsy) in order to know how to process surgical and cytological specimens and to interpret the histological samples taken for microscopic examination, all of which have direct bearing on patient management and clinical outcome. There is no good substitute for the traditional autopsy for the pathologist-in-training. Furthermore and as a result of observational and teaching experience, it is the opinion of the author that the recent additions of virtual autopsy and virtual microscopy to medical school curricula have done and continue to do a disservice to medical students and clinicians-in-training.

Despite the proven importance of the hospital autopsy, the rate of performance has declined to between 5 and 10% over the past 4 decades and even less than 5% in community hospitals [4,5,6]. The reason for the decline is a 3-prong problem: (not enough) money, aversion by clinical practitioners, and lack of promotion by pathology departments [4]. The Joint Commission on Accreditation of Healthcare Organizations (JCAHO) dropped the mandate for hospitals to perform autopsies on all deaths in 1970 although the organization with the support of the American Society for Clinical Pathology (ASCP) has since recommended that hospitals develop criteria for identifying deaths in which an autopsy should be performed [7,8]. Furthermore, Medicare, Medicaid and other insurers do not reimburse hospitals for the cost of performing autopsies. The lack of reimbursement shifts the burden of the cost for autopsy services onto the next-of-kin who may be unable to afford the $2500-plus charge and therefore not request an autopsy or consent to one. However, some hospitals, particularly teaching hospitals, may cover the cost of autopsy services to document a failure of a surgical intervention or treatment related to a clinical trial. Secondly, clinicians' aversion towards the autopsy may stem from fear of litigation for potential autopsy revelations, overreliance on clinical diagnostic test results, or uncertainty about the logistics of obtaining consent for an autopsy to be performed. The time constraints associated with clinical responsibilities and heavy patient loads probably do not help such an aversion. Thirdly, the promotion of the autopsy to clinicians and their trainees seems to have become less of a priority for hospital pathologists whose time is consumed with responsibilities of teaching, research, and service work and since molecular pathology has become an increasingly prominent diagnostic tool. The lack of per-case reimbursement for time-consuming autopsy work is likely an added disincentive.

The consequences of this 3-prong problem of the waning autopsy rate are far-reaching. They include less accurate vital statistical information which is derived from cause-of-death statements upon which epidemiological and clinical research depends. Furthermore, because of the smaller numbers of medical students that are successfully recruited to pursue pathology as a career, the resultant smaller number of pathology residents available to handle casework has led to an increase in the use of pathologist assistants for the processing of surgical specimens and autopsy work. This further detracts from the education of those pathologists-in-training who remain and leaves the impression that processing of surgical tissues and performance of autopsies is superfluous. Those that continue on to hospital-based practice are less equipped to teach as a result of the continual streamlining of training. Clinicians-in-training, who are not required to observe or participate in autopsies, become further removed from understanding the relevance that autopsies have to clinical practice.

Suggestions for improvement of the subpar hospital autopsy rate have been proffered to address the impediments encountered in both clinical and pathology practice, particularly in academic institutions [9]. The creation of multispecialty quality assurance teams inclusive of pathologists and protocols for autopsy performance at regional autopsy centers has been proposed as ways to address educational deficiencies and reduce costs. Optimal scheduling of autopsies to encourage attendance by clinicians and timely completion of autopsy reports that include clear and concise clinicopathologic correlation statements have also been proposed. Importantly, the inclusion of the family regarding the specifics, expectations, and benefits of the autopsy during the terminal stages of an impending death has been suggested in order to make obtaining consent for the performance of an autopsy more feasible. The family should also be provided with upfront information regarding the cost of the autopsy including the possibility of waiving such cost if the death occurred within the teaching hospital or resulted from surgical intervention or treatment occurring during a clinical trial. Where offered, the option of a limited autopsy utilizing molecular diagnostics, computed tomography, or magnetic resonance imaging as adjuncts or supplements to the standard autopsy should be offered to families for consideration, particularly for families with personal or religious objections. It is refreshing to see that the importance and benefits of the autopsy are still genuinely recognized amongst some in clinical practice [10]. It also is fortunate that in many teaching hospitals across the country, the morbidity and mortality conference remains an important educational forum for the review and discussion of medical complications and adverse outcomes in select cases inclusive of relevant anatomic and clinical pathologic findings. It is also a requirement by the Accreditation Council for Graduate Medical Education (ACGME) that all teaching hospitals have regularly scheduled conferences of this type.

Basic differences exist between hospital autopsies and forensic autopsies performed in medical examiner/coroner (ME/C) offices. The aim of the forensic autopsy (also referred to as medical-legal or medicolegal autopsy) in particular is to document the cause of death and the relevant anatomic and clinical pathology components in the context of the death circumstances in a way that will help to answer any questions of legal importance and to facilitate legal proceedings that may follow. This is not the initial aim of a hospital autopsy although it is important to note that at *any* time in the future, well after completion of a hospital autopsy, questions of legal importance may arise stemming from a malpractice or wrongful death claim filed by the family or representative on behalf of the decedent. While the ultimate goal of the hospital autopsy is also to determine the cause of death, a greater emphasis is placed on identifying the anatomic correlate to the signs and symptoms observed and measured during hospitalization.

Further stipulations for the actual autopsy setting and the extent of the autopsy to be performed also apply. In-hospital, non-ME/C deaths may receive an autopsy per request of next-of-kin, which may be limited to a body region. In-hospital deaths under the jurisdiction of the ME/C may receive an autopsy under the direction of the ME/C, which will be a full autopsy. At the ME/C's office, a forensic autopsy will be performed on selected cases, ideally by a trained forensic pathologist or a supervised forensic pathologist-in-training (a fellow), although in some jurisdictions, ME/C autopsies are performed by non-forensic pathologists. In teaching hospitals with anatomic pathology residency training programs, the autopsy is often performed by the pathology resident under the supervision of an attending pathologist. The pathology resident is responsible for obtaining the relevant clinical information from the medical record and/or clinicians and serves as a conduit of communication between the clinicians and attending (supervising) pathologist. Autopsy conferences may be held whereby the pathology resident presents his/her gross findings. When held, these sessions provide an opportunity for clinicians and clinicians-in-training to get instant clinicopathologic correlation on their patients and the information can be relayed to family members with the emphasis that the findings are *preliminary*. The attending pathologist otherwise is responsible for the review of the provisional and final reports compiled and created by the pathology resident, for accuracy and completeness. Both the attending pathologist and pathology resident names will appear on the report with the pathology resident often designated as the **prosector**. In smaller hospitals with autopsy facilities but that lack a pathology residency training program, the attending pathologist will perform all autopsy-related duties. Smaller satellite hospitals lacking autopsy facilities but with affiliations with academic hospitals with such facilities will convey decedents there when an autopsy is warranted.

Whether the autopsy is performed in the hospital or ME/C office setting, it is done following rules and guidelines that govern laboratory safety and universal precautions relative to the utilization of personal protective equipment, handling, retention and disposal of biological material, and maintenance of autopsy-related equipment [11,12]. Adherence to the guidelines and recommendations for standard autopsy practice provided by the College of American Pathologists (CAP) and the National Association of Medical Examiners (NAME) assures high-quality work products [13,14].

5.1 Hospital Autopsies

A death occurring within a medical facility, where the surrounding circumstances do not require medicolegal investigation still may prompt questions regarding the efficacy of medical therapy or accuracy of clinical diagnostic tests to which the autopsy can provide answers and/or clarification. These deaths stem from natural disease with varying degrees and types of therapeutic intervention. The family may express concerns regarding a sudden rapid clinical deterioration ending in death. The autopsy can help allay family concerns and additionally reveal previously unknown disease conditions including those with hereditary implications. Genetic counseling and screening can be offered to relatives of decedents with heritable disease conditions or syndromes revealed by the autopsy. The family can be further reassured by the fact that the autopsy can help the community as a whole through better understanding about the effects of medical treatments which in turn can help future patients. Genetic study of tumor tissue collected during even a limited autopsy can be of great benefit to oncology researchers endeavoring to understand the variation and molecular basis of tumor progression with the ultimate aim to improve clinical diagnosis and treatment thereby reducing morbidity and mortality.

In some instances, the ME/C will assume jurisdiction over a hospital death and allow the autopsy to be performed by or under the direction of the hospital's autopsy pathologist within the hospital. These instances generally entail sudden and unexpected death following a period of hospitalization in those with known chronic natural disease in which there is no suspicion of foul play, trauma, intoxicants or poisons. This may also entail certain deaths in which trauma or intoxicants may be known or suspected and will require additional autopsy documentation, specimen collection and testing. Preliminary and final autopsy reports will be sent to the ME/C and the reports will be reviewed for determination of cause and manner of death and completion of the death certificate. Other ME/C offices utilize local hospital autopsy facilities for the completion of autopsies on all cases for which jurisdiction have been taken, employing either non-forensic pathologists or forensic pathologists.

5.1.1 Consent

Either the clinical practitioner or family may request that an autopsy be performed. The family must be educated as to the goals and procedures of the autopsy as part of the informed consent process and as required by statutes. It should be recognized that the constitution of a family may include traditional and alternative members or otherwise as outlined by the laws of a given locale such as those that apply to domestic partners. They should be reassured that in most cases, the autopsy procedure will not cause disfigurement and that they will be able to have a normal funeral service that includes viewing of their loved one if so desired. Accommodation of families with religious preferences and requirements including timeliness of autopsy completion and handling of the body and bodily fluids must be done. The College of American Pathologists has published a concise and informational brochure that can be provided to families who may be considering an autopsy and need additional, easy-to-understand information or otherwise can be provided as a vehicle of informed consent [15]. Formal written consent for an autopsy must be obtained from the legal next-of-kin, legal representative or healthcare surrogate which will be facilitated by the morgue attendant in larger medical facilities or otherwise directly by the physician or other authorized medical personnel. The consent form serves as an official record to document decedent information, consentee information, autopsy restrictions, and handling of any retained organs and tissues. Appendix F features a sample consent and authorization form adapted from the sample form provided by the College of American Pathologists [16].

5.1.2 History

Knowledge of the medical history is a virtual given when performing a hospital autopsy. This information is readily available from the **electronic medical record (EMR)** or verbally via direct discussion with the clinicians involved in the past or present care of the patient. Particularly in academic hospitals, clinicians and clinicians-in-training are afforded the opportunity to attend autopsies and provide guidance to the prosector and attending pathologist as it pertains to answering questions of clinical importance and during those times have the benefit of receiving instant clinicopathological correlation without having to wait for preliminary or final autopsy reports. This can better equip the clinician with information that can then be relayed to family members in order to keep them up to date and help allay concerns regarding the terminal clinical course of their loved one.

5.1.3 Identification and External Examination

When commencing the hospital autopsy procedure beginning with the external examination, positive identification in many instances has already been established and verified. Upon commencement of the autopsy, additional verification of the patient's identification will be made via comparison of identifying information on the patient's hospital identification bracelet and toe tags with that listed in the medical records. Evidence of surgical or other therapeutic interventions obvious upon external view of the body also serves as an additional basis of comparison to the medical record information. As outlined in the hospital's written policy, procedural efforts to establish the identification of unidentified or unidentifiable patients may be necessary in a few instances and may not have been completed in the case of a death occurring on or shortly after arrival.

The determination of time of death is not an issue as there has been and official pronouncement of the time and date which has been entered into the medical record. As such and unlike in medicolegal or forensic autopsies, assessment of the degree of rigor or livor mortis for the estimation of time of death is not necessary.

The external examination proceeds with a general assessment with description of anatomic features and abnormalities of the nude body after removal of hospital clothing as street clothing is typically not present on the decedent that has had a prolonged hospitalization. Use of a body diagram to document external changes such as therapeutic devices, scars, injuries, and lesions is common while photographic documentation may or may not accompany diagrammatic description. Special collection of foreign material as evidence is not part of the routine hospital autopsy. Pre-death, in-hospital collection of trace evidence may be performed by or at the direction of a law enforcement officer or, in cases involving sexual assault, a forensically-trained clinical practitioner. Imaging studies already performed in the antemortem period generally will not be repeated in the postmortem period and may not have been performed in the case of death on arrival or death occurring within a short time after arrival to the hospital following cessation of resuscitative efforts. The exception to this would be in the instance that postmortem computed tomography or magnetic resonance imaging studies have been performed at facilities with designated equipment and protocols already in place.

If unusual external findings inconsistent with therapeutic intervention and suggestive of something other than natural disease changes are encountered, reporting of the death to the ME/C will follow. Optimally, this will be promptly communicated to the attending clinician of record who must then notify the family or legal representative so that they can update their chosen funeral home as necessary.

5.1.4 Internal Examination

The extent of the examination of the internal organs and tissues will depend on the stipulations on the consent form such as permission to examine the brain only (with or without spinal cord), chest organs only, chest and abdominal organs only, abdominopelvic organs only, or all of the organs. The total time to completion of the autopsy will vary and depend on these stipulations in addition to the complexity of the autopsy and the experience of the prosecting pathologist. Organs may be removed and fixed in formalin for later examination and dissection which can add additional time for completion of the autopsy.

The examination of the internal organs is facilitated by the pathologist assistant who performs the initial Y-incision over the chest and abdominal region with removal of the chest plate and evisceration of the chest and abdominal organs following in situ inspection by the pathologist. If indicated, the brain will be accessed after incision of the scalp with removal of the skull cap and the spinal cord will be accessed via anterior or posterior dissection of the spine, prior to removal. Removal of implantable devices like pacemakers, defibrillators, muscle stimulators, and medication pumps, is done to prevent hazards that may occur during cremation. These devices may also be retained by protocol or at the request of the next-of-kin, the manufacturer of the device, insurance companies, or attorneys, particularly if concerns of malfunction are raised. Photographic documentation of gross pathological changes of the viscera both in situ and upon dissection is performed more often than that of the external body and often more so for educational purposes. All examined organs may be retained and not returned to the body unless further stipulated by the autopsy consent form.

Routinely, histological samples are obtained and submitted for processing by a histotechnologist for later review and interpretation by the pathologist. Samples of bodily fluids like blood, urine, and bile may be collected for temporary storage or for submission for serological and biochemical analysis. Collection for clinical toxicological analyses of therapeutic drugs may also be done. Sampling of abscesses, abnormal fluid collections, and tissues for microbial and viral testing may be done. In sepsis-related deaths in which the origin remains unclear, devices such as catheters and arteriovenous fistulas may also be cultured for microbial testing.

If unusual findings inconsistent with the clinical presentation or course or otherwise suggestive of non-natural entities such as trauma or drug overdose are encountered during the external and internal examination, the autopsy will be halted with subsequent notification made to the ME/C. If jurisdiction is assumed, any samples of bodily fluids that were obtained during the autopsy will be sent along with the body to the ME/C's office. The hospital pathology department may also have a pre-established protocol that directs the collection of blood, urine, bile, gastric and ocular (vitreous) fluids on cases in which the ME/C has assumed jurisdiction.

5.1.5 Postmortem Testing and Clinical Correlates

In hospital autopsies, the collection of blood, urine, CSF, and tissues for chemistry testing and microbial cultures is done with frequency as dictated by the clinical presentation and/or hospital course. By contrast, the collection of bodily fluids like blood and urine specifically for postmortem toxicology testing is performed infrequently, and generally not on a routine basis. The opportunity to investigate a death suspected to have resulted from overmedication, undermedication, or intake of illicit substances while hospitalized thus cannot be fully undertaken, especially in the case of prolonged hospitalization where the earlier blood and urine samples may have already been discarded. This is a well-recognized limitation relative to forensic autopsies. Illicit drug- or medication-associated deaths must be reported to the ME/C regardless of the unavailability of certain specimens.

It may be difficult to establish or confirm a suspected intoxication in a decedent who has had a prolonged hospitalization due to the unavailability of specimens obtained on admission or in the early period of hospitalization. Review of results of *any* antemortem testing for illicit drugs and other intoxicants alongside baseline changes in the patient's clinical status may be helpful. Even with the availability of specimens for testing, it is important for clinicians to recognize the limitations of hospital-based screening of blood and urine for the presence of illicit drugs and intoxicants [17,18].

Urine drug screening (UDS) is a two-step process involving an immunoassay screen and confirmatory screening of positive results using a different method such as gas chromatography-mass spectrometry (GC-MS). This screening modality has been automated allowing quick turnaround time so vital to patient management. A urine drug screen may have been performed shortly after admission and reported as positive, indicative of an acute intoxication or historic drug/medication use. Results reported as negative may represent the true absence of a drug or medication, or more precisely that there was no detection of drugs or medications **targeted by the actual test panel used in the laboratory**. Furthermore, a negative screen result does not guarantee complete absence of a suspected drug or medication as many test panels have a pre-determined threshold limit of detection for each drug or medication targeted whereby if the concentration is below that limit, the result will be reported as negative. Similarly, a positive screen result is not a guarantee for the presence of a particular substance as it could also indicate consumption of a structurally similar medication, drug, or food substance that cross-reacts with the test giving rise to a false positive result. A positive screen result may also represent pre- or in-hospital administration of certain medications which warrants clinical correlation. A positive UDS test should prompt the clinician to request confirmatory testing by an alternate method such as GC-MS. The frequency of use or dosing, status of hydration, pH of the urine, pharmacogenetics, pharmacogenomics, half-life, and volume of distribution are additional factors that can affect whether or not a drug or medication and its metabolites are detected in the urine. Clinical symptomatology suggestive of intoxication should prompt further testing on blood inclusive of send-out testing for substances that may have been missed on the UDS, along with institution of empirical therapy in order to mitigate clinical complications [19].

A drug/medication screen on admission *blood* may also have been performed, which is a better indicator of acute toxicity, but again, only for the drugs and medications covered in the panel. Furthermore, many of the factors affecting detection of drugs and medications in urine also apply to blood. Glycols, like ethylene glycol and propylene glycol are not included in typical urine and blood screen panels and therefore a specific request to test for these substances must be done and empirical therapy initiated promptly if clinically suspected [20]. Another example is fentanyl, which despite having similar effects on the body, it is chemically distinct from other opiates and opioids and therefore will not be detected by the standard test panels used in many hospital laboratories. Patients presenting as and later dying from a presumed heroin overdose and treated as such have later been found on postmortem testing performed in forensic toxicology laboratories to have died as a result of fentanyl or combined heroin and fentanyl overdose. Moreover, a myriad of obscure, clandestinely synthesized, highly potent and rapidly fatal drug and medication analogues known as Novel Psychoactive Substances (NPS) are not detected by the standard screening test kits used in hospitals [21].

In all cases with clinical suspicion of overdose or intoxication, it is prudent for clinicians to know or find out the scope of the screening test panel used in their hospital or hospital-affiliated laboratory, including the limits of analyte detection, sensitivities, specificities, and cross-reactions, by communication with laboratory personnel. Consultation with a clinical pathologist or medical toxicologist may also be necessary towards that aim which may prompt the submission of samples to outside reference laboratories for identification of substances not tested for in-house. Similarly, the hospital autopsy pathologist must also be cognizant of the limitations of not only clinical toxicological testing but also recognize the limitations of postmortem toxicology testing discussed further in section 5.2.6.

5.1.6 Reporting

Reporting of findings is standard for hospital autopsies and includes a list of **preliminary or provisional anatomic diagnoses (PAD).** The PAD report is followed sometime later by a list of the **final anatomic diagnoses (FAD**) after review and interpretation of postmortem test results such as microbial cultures and prepared histological sections. The list of anatomic diagnoses is often accompanied by a list of clinical pathological diagnoses documented during hospitalization organized by organ system. chronologically, or by order of importance based on the severity of the anatomic and/or clinical pathological findings. Any restrictions stipulated on the autopsy consent form will affect the comprehensiveness of the PAD or FAD. Other standard components of what will become the FAD report are the medical record number, demographic data, a summary of the clinical history, description of the organ systems, microscopic description/diagnosis of sectioned tissues, ancillary findings (serological, cytogenetic, electron microscopic, molecular diagnostic, and histochemical results) and a clinicopathologic summary statement that ties together the antemortem clinical information with the postmortem findings inclusive of a statement of the cause of death. Reference to results stemming from antemortem surgical pathology, cytopathology, and clinical pathology examinations inclusive of alphanumeric accessioning numbers are routinely included.

If organized by order of importance, the first item or section listed in the FAD and sometimes the PAD often includes the major anatomic or clinical pathological diagnosis incompatible with life and therefore some version of that item should be included in the cause-of-death statement on the death certificate. Alternatively, a chronological listing of clinical and pathological findings from earliest to the latest, inclusive of terminal mechanism(s) and pathophysiological derangements ending in death may be done and thus the *last* item or section is an important component of the cause of death and some form of this should appear on the death certificate.

It is imperative that the attending pathologist and attending clinician (or the designated authorized person who will complete the death certificate) come to a consensus and understanding through discussion as to the most probable, etiologically specific cause of death based on the anatomic and clinical pathological findings. If it is anticipated by the attending pathologist that major FAD findings will substantially differ from the PAD findings, this should be promptly communicated to the certifying clinician who at that time should also be instructed to enter the word *"pending"* in the cause-of-death section on the death certificate initially. Upon receipt of the FAD autopsy report inclusive of the clinicopathologic summary and cause-of-death statements some time later, the appropriate, etiologically specific final cause of death can then be entered on the supplemental or final death certificate. This may be necessary since most states require the completion of the death certificate within a few days which most likely will be before final autopsy results become available. Otherwise, if the certifying clinician has already certified the death based on provisional findings and the FAD findings differ significantly, the attending pathologist must notify the certifying clinician, discuss the findings, and request that an amended death certificate be issued. Furthermore, **it is incumbent upon the certifying clinician to be mindful and anticipate that the findings of the autopsy (preliminary or final) are forthcoming and initiate or maintain an open line of communication with the pathologist to ensure that the most accurate and etiologically specific cause of death will appear on the death certificate, one that is consistent with or preferably the same as that contained in the PAD and/or FAD reports**. Consistency is important because discrepancies between the cause of death listed on the autopsy report and the cause of death listed on the death certificate can be problematic for anyone who has obtained and reviewed copies of both documents such as family members, insurance companies, attorneys, risk management officers, researchers, and epidemiologists. Medical facilities may find it preferable and advantageous for the attending pathologist who performed or supervised the autopsy to certify the death, after consultation with the attending physician.

The autopsy report contains identifying and detailed medical information and becomes part of the patient's medical record which is protected by federal law as outlined in the Health Insurance Portability and Accountability Act (HIPAA).

Accordingly, it is not a public record and copies are provided upon request and at cost to the legal next-of-kin or legal representative. Hospital laboratory and medical record information systems allow electronic indexing and retrieval based on alphanumerical and diagnostic identifiers contained in the reports which also become a permanent part of the decedent's medical record. Guidelines and recommendations for standard hospital/medical autopsy performance and reporting are reviewed, revised and published periodically [13]. A sample hospital autopsy report with case scenario information appears in Appendix G.

5.2 Medicolegal/Forensic Autopsies

The ultimate goal of the medicolegal or forensic autopsy is to determine the cause and manner of death with completion of the death certificate. This entails deaths occurring under violent or otherwise unnatural circumstances as outlined in the recommendations of the 1954 Model Postmortem Examination Act, adopted in most US jurisdictions and outlined in varying degree in the statutes [22]. Information generated from medicolegal/forensic autopsies is additionally for the education and benefit of the community as a whole and its subsections including lay, legal, and medical constituents in regards to matters of health and safety. The performance of a medicolegal or forensic autopsy is considered a practice of medicine and is best performed by a board-certified or board-eligible forensic pathologist or a supervised pathologist-in-training [23]. Surprisingly, this is required by law in only 20 states and the District of Columbia [24].

The autopsy procedure itself is but one component of a medicolegal autopsy. Analysis of the death scene and history, laboratory analysis of fluids and tissues collected during the autopsy, and the utilization of ancillary procedures and expertise are other important components (Table 5.1). In addition to cause and manner-of-death determination, the medicolegal autopsy strives to answer 5 important questions:

- Who is the decedent? (verify or establish identification)
- Where did the decedent die? (death scene information)
- When did the decedent die? (time of death, postmortem interval)
- How did the decedent die? (disease, injury, intoxication/poisoning, or combination)

- What were the circumstances surrounding the death? (natural vs. non-natural, manner of death)

Undiagnosed disease including cancers, infections, endocrine complications, and heritable disease syndromes are sometimes found at autopsy to be the cause of death. Certain disease findings that may have a genetic basis could have important health implications for the surviving blood relatives and it is within the purview of the forensic pathologist to recommend discussion with a primary care provider regarding referral for genetic counseling and screening services.

ME/C autopsy services are for the benefit of the public and do not incur additional costs to families, estates, or the citizenry as the services are pre-paid with tax dollars.

5.2.1 Consent

While the statutes require identification of the legal next-of-kin for notification purposes, they do not require informed consent from next-of kin for the performance of a medicolegal autopsy, one fundamental difference between hospital autopsies. Furthermore, the medicolegal autopsy is not restricted to body regions and generally a full autopsy with examination of most or all of the major organs will be performed. Organs and tissues, whole are part, may be retained for testing and research purposes, as outlined in the statutes. Certain restrictions may apply as it pertains to religious preferences including rules and rites governing the handling of the body and bodily fluids and the time within which the autopsy must be completed so as not to hinder or delay religious proceedings. There may be a religious objection to the performance of an autopsy altogether and any objection is discussed and addressed within the context of the legal responsibilities of the ME/C, particularly if the death is homicidal. The medical examiner or coroner is wise to initiate and maintain open lines of communication with the heads of the local religious communities as it pertains to their beliefs and practices regarding autopsies.

5.2.2 History

In contrast to the hospital setting, it is common for historical information including medical history to be incomplete or unknown altogether. Medicolegal death investigators responding to deaths occurring outside of a medical facility will make diligent efforts to locate and inventory any medications, document any use of medical devices, obtain any medical paperwork, and obtain a verbal history from family members and acquaintances, all of which are vital to the forensic pathologist. However, such items and history may be unavailable particularly if the decedent was socially isolated or had not been under medical care for a period of time prior to death.

Incomplete or absent medical history poses a unique challenge to the practice of forensic pathology in which the experienced practitioner learns to adopt an anticipatory mindset as to the varied possibilities regarding the cause of death and adapt the autopsy procedure accordingly. Review of medical records is an essential component of the medicolegal autopsy, particularly if a medical facility was the place of death, as this is akin to the death scene. Even though electronic medical records are well-established in many hospitals and their affiliated facilities, many ME/C offices do not have access to them although this is slowly changing. Paper copies are often obtained but initially may be sparse. Often, upon commencing the autopsy, the forensic pathologist may have only the emergency medical services run report, a few pages of the emergency department or admission records, the hospital's summary report to the coroner or medical examiner, or no such records at all. Additional records are often received later after the autopsy has been completed. Many of the hospital records, especially the narratives containing interpretations of diagnostic data and procedures or regarding the patient's clinical status, are initially unavailable because they have not been dictated, transcribed or otherwise electronically entered. Before, during, or after the autopsy, the forensic pathologist will seek any additional medical records necessary including admission and discharge summaries, radiology reports, operative reports, and laboratory/toxicology reports.

The forensic pathologist may also contact the treating clinician directly, before commencing an autopsy procedure to inquire about the medical history and the type and extent of medical intervention(s) not found in the medical records initially received but otherwise evident on external or internal examination. In gunshot wound cases with surgical intervention, the surgeon may be called to find out the number, condition, and anatomic location of any projectiles recovered during surgery and the disposition of the same as this is relevant to the number of entry and exit wounds found at autopsy. Inquiry regarding the placement and removal of chest tubes including the quantity and type of fluid drained, whether wounds were surgical or inflicted, and whether any inflicted wounds were utilized as access ports may be made. Accurate documentation of penetrating torso wounds caused by objects such as bullets and knives is of utmost forensic importance for investigative reasons and for potential future court proceedings. Craniectomy specimens with defects produced by bullets will be especially sought after because certain characteristics of the defect convey specific information regarding direction of travel of the bullet and the proximity of the firearm to the head upon discharge.

Review of police reports inclusive of photographs prior to the autopsy or verbal communication with law enforcement officers regarding death scene findings are also commonly done. Law enforcement officers may also attend autopsies, particularly homicidal cases, and convey important death scene information. Other non-hospital records may be obtained and reviewed such as child and adult protective service reports, engineering reports, traffic/crash reports, fire reports, and incident reports from the workplace, group home, or jail.

5.2.3 Identification

Decedent identification is an absolute requirement in medicolegal death investigation not only for proper death certification and for the families but also for the investigation by law enforcement of deaths involving foul play. Thus, ultimately it is necessary in order to prevent the miscarriage of justice in certain cases. Not uncommonly, a decedent may arrive unidentified or tentatively identified for many reasons such as the death was unwitnessed, estrangement from family members, disfiguring injuries, decompositional changes or lack of identification cards. Regardless of the condition of the body, photographic documentation of the face (identification photograph) and the overall body is done upon receiving the body into the ME/C's facility. Presumptive identification is aided by certain physical characteristics, tattoos, type of clothing, and jewelry which family members can be shown via viewing of photographs taken at the

ME/C's office or direct viewing of the body. Engraved jewelry and dentures are other items sought and used as presumptive identifiers. Identification by scientific methods will promptly follow via fingerprinting, dental charting with comparison to antemortem images, and DNA comparison to profiles stored in databases or to profiles obtained from blood relatives. Prostheses and implantable devices like pacemakers and defibrillators commonly have serial numbers and other manufacturer information inscribed on them which are also recorded in the patient's medical record at the time of implantation. These devices can be examined in situ or removed entirely at the time of the autopsy in order to obtain the identifiers and use them as a basis for identification by comparison to recorded information in the medical record of the suspected individual. Surgical tissues retained in pathology departments are a source of DNA which can be compared to DNA obtained from the decedent during autopsy. Droplets of blood placed on filter paper, buccal swabs, and hair with roots are commonly obtained during autopsy as DNA standards and retained in storage in case they are needed later to establish or confirm identity or to establish or confirm parentage or relationship. Antemortem and postmortem radiographic comparisons of unique skeletal attributes such as the configuration of the craniofacial sinuses and spinal osteophytes can be made and utilized for identification. Even the number and configuration of the twists of sternotomy wires and the number and placement of surgical clips related to remote coronary artery bypass grafting can be used as a basis for identification via comparison of antemortem and postmortem radiographs. Antemortem radiographs are commonly available in digital format and can be sent to the pathologist either on a storage device or electronically. For decedents arriving from the hospital, verification of the identification by comparison of hospital identification bracelets and toe tags with the medical record information will be done in all cases. Badly decomposed, charred, or skeletonized bodies are inherently unrecognizable and will require the expertise of the forensic (DNA) scientist, forensic anthropologist, and forensic odontologist to assist in the identification process. When the initial efforts towards identification are exhausted, it will become necessary to widen the scope and obtain additional assistance starting with registering the decedent on national databases such as the National Missing and Unidentified Persons System (NamUs) (https://namus.gov).

5.2.4 External Examination

Certain death circumstances will dictate performance of pre-autopsy forensic scientific examinations, in stark contrast to hospital cases. Homicidal, suicidal, some accidental, and otherwise suspicious deaths warrant careful examination before any further manipulation related to autopsy procedures or tissue procurement is done. Badly decomposed bodies colonized by insects or plant material may warrant expert examination by a forensic entomologist or botanist. Examination of skeletal remains requires the expertise of the forensic anthropologist and, with recovery of the maxilla and mandible, the forensic odontologist. In certain cases, especially homicides, the forensic scientist will examine the body and perform trace evidence collection from clothing or directly form the skin surface sometimes utilizing microscopy or an alternate light source such as ultraviolet light as guides. A chemical spray may be applied directly to clothing with defects from bullets to facilitate detection of gunpowder residue in order to assist in range-of-fire determination. Examination of clothing (especially undergarments), pubic hair combings, swabs from body surfaces, cavities, and bitemarks for the presence of foreign DNA are done in deaths involving or suspected to involve sexual violence. Any clothing on the body is removed prior to the autopsy. In certain cases, like homicides, the clothing will be retained as evidence and further examined. Otherwise the clothing will be released along with the body to the funeral home.

ME/C cases involving penetrating injuries, pedestrian accidents, child abuse, decomposition, charred, and skeletonized remains warrant radiological examination prior to autopsy. Recovery of evidence, determination of identity, and determination of antemortem skeletal injury is all aided by this ancillary procedure. Radiological examination facilitates the localization of retained foreign material like bullets, fracture patterns, and implantable devices prior to dissection and reduces unnecessary and prolonged dissection. Modalities such as x-ray, computed tomography (CT), and magnetic resonance imaging (MRI) are used variably at ME/C offices. CT and MRI scanners are not available at all offices due to infrastructure and budgetary constraints and the inadequate numbers of personnel with specialized training in forensic radiology.

After completion of ancillary, pre-autopsy tasks, further external examination of the body performed by the forensic pathologist is the next important part of the medicolegal autopsy. Upon receipt of the decedent into the

ME/C's facility, the body is first weighed, photographed, and measured for height and general identifying characteristics are recorded. After these features along with the assigned case number and other identifiers are verified, careful attention is turned to the description of injuries, therapeutic devices, scars, and identifying features like tattoos, with inclusion of anatomic reference points and measurements in a least 2 dimensions, head to toe, front and back. Documentation with clinical correlation of resuscitative injuries such as chest abrasions, burns from defibrillation pads, and ecchymosis caused by venipunctures is important. Identification of stigmata of chronic drug use will guide postmortem toxicological testing. The quality and quantity of fluids draining from the body orifices provide clues to the underlying cause of death. Examples include residual food material within the oral cavity in choking deaths, hematochezia associated with deaths due to gastrointestinal hemorrhage, or the presence of a foam cone in opiate deaths. Deformity and asymmetry of limbs will be documented and may indicate congenital abnormalities or skeletal injury and may warrant radiological examination prior to continuation of the autopsy. The use of annotated body diagrams to depict external changes is common as well as photographic documentation of the same.

Identification with documentation of postmortem and other skin changes is standard and can be of forensic importance in non-natural deaths. The degree of **rigor mortis** and the location and appearance of **livor mortis** is assessed carefully as the characteristics and qualities of these changes provide information not only about the **time of death (TOD)** and the position of the body at death but also activity at death (i.e. cadaveric spasm) and signs of poisoning (i.e. cherry red lividity with carbon monoxide poisoning). Faint lividity, pale mucosae, and pale nail beds may indicate acute blood loss or chronic anemia. Decompositional changes such as bloating, marbling, and skin slippage are factors in the estimation of not only the TOD but also the time elapsed after death prior to examination of the body, known as the **postmortem interval (PMI)**. The appearance and distribution of skin discolorations provides clues to underlying pathology or injury. For instance, the location and distribution of petechial hemorrhage can be the difference between the diagnosis of manual strangulation (facial and conjunctival petechiae) or disseminated intravascular coagulation caused by meningococcemia (diffuse petechiae) and affect the direction and focus of the rest of the autopsy.

The external examination in deaths due to penetrating or blunt force injuries is often as important as or more important than the internal examination.

In a homicidal gunshot wound case, documenting the location of entrance wounds and any exit wounds, the direction of the bullet upon entry, and information as to how far the gun was away from the body at the time it was fired (range of fire) and sometimes the position of the victim relative to the assailant, is vital to law enforcement officers who are tasked with reconstructing the circumstances surrounding the death. The accurate description and detailed documentation in a homicidal blunt force injury case can provide important information to law enforcement in their search for the object used to assault the victim or to corroborate death scene findings of a struggle. The pattern and distribution of blunt force injuries on a pedestrian victim of a hit-skip automobile accident can provide clues to investigators regarding evasive maneuvers or contact with the various surfaces of the vehicle. Any visible foreign materials will be collected by the forensic pathologist or directly by the forensic scientist at the direction of the forensic pathologist and submitted to the appropriate laboratory according to chain-of-custody protocol. Photograph documentation of all injuries of significance, before and after any cleaning away of blood and debris or removal of therapeutic devices, is standard practice in medicolegal autopsies.

Just as it is important to photograph injuries and other positive findings, documentation of pertinent negatives can be just as important or even more important. For example, if the death scene and historical information or an alleged witness account indicated that a death involved manual strangulation, but the autopsy examination did not reveal changes consistent with the history and statements, then photographic documentation of the external and internal neck regions lacking skin contusions, strap muscle hemorrhages, and fracture of the hyoid bone and thyroid cartilage all constitute pertinent negatives.

5.2.5 Internal Examination

As with hospital autopsies, the internal examination begins with the Y-incision over the chest and abdomen with subsequent removal of the chest plate and evisceration of the chest and abdominal organs, after in situ inspection. Identification of subgaleal injury upon reflection of the scalp is of particular importance when assessing for blunt impact head injury since oftentimes external scalp injury is not visible or is otherwise hidden by hair. Removal of the skull cap with subsequent removal of the brain, after in situ inspection, will follow which importantly includes stripping of the dura to reveal any fractures that could be hidden beneath. The gross examination of the axial and appendicular skeleton is done and at times with the guidance of pre-autopsy imaging results. The standard medicolegal autopsy is a full autopsy with examination of all of the major organs with a few exceptions and as dictated by the type of case. For example, the spinal cord and the laryngotracheal complex may not be removed in all cases. Furthermore, retained foreign materials such as bullets constitute evidence and will be recovered and submitted according to chain-of-custody protocol to the appropriate forensic laboratory.

Specialized dissections focused on documenting or ruling out certain injuries may also be performed in medicolegal autopsies which are not done in hospital autopsies. Dissection of the anterior neck with layer-by-layer reflection and examination of the cervical strap muscles and the underlying larnygotracheal complex is done in cases of manual or ligature strangulation. Removal of the laryngotracheal complex in continuity with the tongue is done in deaths possibly due to choking, seizures, or involving injury to this region. In infant deaths from suspected inflicted craniocerebral injury, the eyes and attached optic nerve will be removed for examination for retinal hemorrhages. Craniocerebral arteries may be accessed for injection using contrast material and imaged in cases of suspected trauma leading to stroke. Deaths due to iatrogenic introduction of air into the cavities or associated with underwater diving warrant specialized dissections to assess for pneumothorax or air embolism. As in hospital autopsies, examination of the veins of the lower and sometimes upper extremities will be performed after the discovery of a pulmonary arterial thromboembolus. Dissection of limbs to document fractures revealed by pre-autopsy imaging may be needed in order to assist in the estimation of the timing of the injury.

Tissue sections from major organs, lesions, and injuries are obtained and submitted in formalin for histological preparation. Particularly, microscopic examination of skin, visceral injuries, and fracture sites is of medicolegal importance as it can reveal the presence of foreign material of evidentiary value or provide evidence of a survival interval prior to death. Injury, if sustained during life, often causes hemorrhage which leads to inflammation and the subsequent stages of healing. This is also known as **vital reaction,** an important marker of survival, however brief, after injury. The elucidation of pulmonary pathology associated with chronic drug or medication abuse by inhalational and intravenous routes gives insight into the history and direction for postmortem toxicological testing. Histological evidence of diabetic nephropathy will prompt postmortem testing for metabolic complications of diabetes mellitus if not already done so based on the medical history. Suspected hematological disease may prompt preparation of peripheral smears for special staining. The number of sections obtained varies by the type of case. In some ME/C offices certain cases such as gunshot wound and hanging cases may have very little if any histological sampling performed. Sampling with submission of blood and tissues for microbial analysis in suspected cases of sepsis or organ-based infection may be performed. Sampling of purulent fluid collections from body cavities or tissues with submission for microbial analysis is routinely performed and can yield organism-specific results pertinent to the cause of death.

Smaller portions of major organs, glands, and bone are retained in a stock jar containing formalin for a few years duration prior to medical disposal. Rarely, it may be necessary to return to the archived tissue to obtain additional sections for microscopic examination. The remainder of the unsampled organs is returned to the decedent's body cavity to accompany the body to the funeral home for final disposition. Retention of whole organs with fixation in formalin for later dissection may be required in certain cases which is either permitted by state law or requires permission from the legal next-of-kin.

Implantable devices such as pacemakers, implantable cardioverter defibrillators (ICDs), and insulin pumps are accessed, inspected in situ, descriptively and/or photographically documented, and removed from the body as they may present potential hazards should the body be later cremated. They may be retained indefinitely or returned with the decedent's belongings. Outside technicians may be called upon to interrogate devices like ICDs when a cardiac death is suspected or a cardiac event is suspected to have precipitated injury both of which are of medicolegal importance should questions later arise concerning manufacturing defects or liability in personal injury cases. Information obtained from ICDs have been shown to be instrumental in the determination of the time of injury and the TOD [25]. Similarly, examination of medication pumps may be warranted to rule out under- or overmedication associated with device malfunction. Retention of medical devices may be warranted particularly if it is known that such devices have been reported to the U.S. Food and Drug Administration's MedWatch program, as further investigation may necessitate examination of the actual device.

Uncomplicated autopsies such as drug overdoses in young individuals or deaths due to cardiac diseases may take approximately an hour to complete. Complicated autopsies such as deaths due to multiple gunshot wounds, homicidal blunt force injury deaths, or skeletonized remains may take hours or days to complete due to various ancillary examinations and collections that may be necessary. Next-day examination in homicidal blunt force injury deaths is at times necessary as certain injuries are often more visible after organs have been removed and much of the confounding blood has drained out of the vasculature. All external and internal findings are descriptively, photographically, and diagrammatically documented to varying degrees as dictated by the type of case.

5.2.6 Postmortem Testing

The collection and submission of bodily fluids and tissues for postmortem testing is routine and standard practice in medicolegal or forensic autopsies. *The postmortem forensic toxicology laboratory is responsible for the qualitative and quantitative analysis of submitted specimens for drugs of abuse, medications, electrolytes and osmolytes in order to aid the forensic pathologist in the determination of the cause of death, contributing factor(s) in the death, and the manner of death.* Deaths known or suspected to be the result of motor vehicle accidents, drug use, fires, homicidal violence, suicide, over- or undermedication, poisoning, metabolic complications of disease, or infection require postmortem testing. As necessary and importantly, any available hospital admission blood and urine samples will be obtained and submitted for testing in the postmortem forensic toxicology laboratory which generally is more comprehensive than the standard screening tests done in hospitals, with the exception of ethanol testing and therapeutic drug monitoring. Results of testing on antemortem specimens can be compared to those obtained from testing on postmortem specimens to help determine if the intoxication occurred prior to the terminal admission or during hospitalization and the degree of metabolism if any.

Collection of central blood (heart), peripheral blood (femoral vein), vitreous fluid, urine, gastric contents, and bile is routine. Variably, fat, muscle, cerebral spinal fluid, and solid organ tissues are also collected. Abundant sample quantity is usually the rule except in infants and in cases of extreme exsanguination and decomposition. Even in the early postmortem period, changes in sample quality mediated by intracellular enzymes (autolysis) and bacteria (putrefaction) occur. Hemolysis also occurs. Certain blood enzymes like blood esterases remain active after death and continue to metabolize certain drugs in vivo. All of these changes cause degradation of specimens with loss of analytes including drugs of abuse like cocaine, production of ethanol by the fermentation process, and production of putrefactive amines similar to amphetamines. In severely decomposed cases, specimen degradation is pronounced and will severely limit or preclude analyte detection or yield results of little value for interpretation. Preservation of postmortem samples is thus necessary to prevent or retard these changes. This is aided by the addition of an antibacterial sodium fluoride and an anticoagulant potassium oxalate. (Note that these chemicals are also contained in blood collection tubes used by hospitals and serve the same purposes.) Refrigeration and freezing of fluid and tissue specimens is also utilized for short- and long-term storage of specimens, respectively in order to prevent of retard degradation.

In contrast to serological testing in the clinical setting, the scope of postmortem serological testing may be limited due to loss or degradation of some serological markers as a result of decomposition and hemolysis, such as enzyme markers for liver damage. Other markers are stable in the early postmortem period and the detection of these markers may be key in the determination of the cause of death. Examples of these include thyroxine measured in the workup of a death due to Grave's disease and tryptase with Immunoglobulin E testing for the workup of an anaphylactic death. Blood collected in red top tubes is submitted for serological testing as necessary.

In certain cases, additional collection and submission for either in-house or outside laboratory testing is necessary. Deaths suspected to result from inhalation of toxic vapors and gases require collection of tracheal aspirates, lung and other tissues for head space chromatography analysis. Hair and nails are collected in certain cases of poisoning such as those involving heavy metals. Blood will be collected into royal blue top tubes in suspected heavy metal poisoning as well. In deaths suspected to be as a result of bacterial or fungal infection, swabs of lung, spleen, abscesses, effusions, and purulent exudates will be done and blood will be collected into aerobic and anaerobic culture bottles, within the recommended 24-hour postmortem time period after death. Cerebral spinal fluid may be obtained and submitted for bacterial or viral analysis by culture or polymerase chain reaction (PCR) testing. Swabs or tissue collection from the airway or lungs may be collected and submitted for viral testing. Blood may be collected and submitted for viral hepatitis and immunodeficiency viral and related antigen markers. Collection of blood spots for metabolic screening is routinely done on cases of sudden death in infants. Sudden deaths in children and adults may warrant collection and submission of blood for genetic testing for hypertrophic cardiomyopathy and the cardiac channelopathies such as Long-QT syndrome and catecholaminergic polymorphous ventricular tachycardia (CPVT).

Immunological-based assays, chromatography, and mass spectrometry are technologies commonly used in postmortem forensic toxicology laboratories. Turn-around-time for in-house toxicological and chemistry testing is variable taking as little as a few days for qualitative screen-based testing up to approximately 6-8 weeks for comprehensive quantitative testing and reporting. Samples may be sent to forensic toxicology reference laboratories which have large-scale testing capabilities with shorter, more predictable turn-around-times.

5.2.7 Reporting

By law, the ME/C is required to keep records of all deaths investigated. Preliminary reports generally are not issued by ME/C offices and only the official final report is generated. Rarely, an amended report may be generated to reflect important changes. The final autopsy report, sometimes referred to the **autopsy protocol**, has several components, with some overlap with that contained within a hospital autopsy report. Consistently, the case number (akin to the hospital medical record number), decedent identifying demographic information, and the date and the time of the commencement of the autopsy are included. Variably, the names of the autopsy assistant and any observers may be included. Provision of a summary page listing the anatomic diagnoses along with the cause and manner of death is customary. A more detailed description of the external body including scars and tattoos, therapeutic interventions and devices, injuries, and recovery of foreign material follows the summary page. Description of findings by organ system inclusive of normal or unremarkable findings is standard. Toxicological findings may be part of the autopsy report itself or a separate document. Reports from some offices include an opinion statement correlating the death circumstances with the autopsy and laboratory findings and otherwise the rationale behind the cause and manner-of-death determination. In some offices, a summary of the circumstances surrounding and leading to the death with reference to emergency medical and law enforcement records, hospital records and the cause and manner of death is created and is known as the **autopsy verdict**. Signatures of the forensic pathologist and chief medical examiner or coroner along with the date of report completion also appear.

Many jurisdictions restrict public access to part or all of the autopsy report including autopsy photographs. In other jurisdictions, the autopsy report with or without autopsy photographs is a public record and subject to request by various constituents of the public. Ancillary reports resulting from examination of evidence are generally separate from the autopsy report and public access is restricted. All reports are stored in paper and/or electronic format. Upon a formal public records request where permitted by statute, copies of unrestricted reports are made available, usually at a nominal cost. If the decedent was hospitalized upon death, it is customary for the ME/C's office to send a copy of the autopsy report to the medical records division of the hospital for inclusion in the medical record. Otherwise, the hospital will request a copy of the report for inclusion in the patient's medical record.

While the autopsy report contains the cause and manner of death which also appears on the death certificate, it is not interchangeable with the death certificate. The death certificate is a separately generated legal document that contains the cause and manner of death determined by the ME/C or designated authorized individual such as a forensic pathologist. Table 5.2 provides a side-by-side comparison of the key differentiating features of hospital and medicolegal autopsies.

Table 5.1 Key Components and Personnel in Medicolegal Autopsies

Component	**Personnel**
Analysis of scene/history	Law Enforcement Emergency Response/Rescue Teams Medical First Responders (i.e. EMS) Medicolegal Death Investigator Forensic Pathologist Forensic Scientist/Anthropologist
External/Internal Examination	Forensic Pathologist Forensic Scientist Pathologist Assistant Forensic Photographer
Collection/Processing/Analysis of bodily fluids and tissues	Forensic Pathologist Pathologist Assistant Histotechnologist Forensic Toxicologist/Drug Chemist
Ancillary Examinations: **Radiological (X-ray, CT, MRI)** **Digital Imaging** **Trace Evidence** **Examination of Skeletonized Remains** **Examination of Colonized Remains**	 Forensic Pathologist/ Radiologist Forensic Photographer Forensic Scientist (Trace Evidence, DNA) Forensic Anthropologist/ Odontologist Forensic Entomologist/Botanist

Table 5.2 Essential Differences between Hospital and Medicolegal/Forensic Autopsies

	Hospital	**Medicolegal**
Overall focus	Cause of death Clinicopathologic correlation	Cause and manner of death Resolution of legal matters
Cost	$2500+, not covered by insurance	Pre-paid for by taxes
Who performs	Hospital pathologist, resident	Forensic or non-forensic pathologist, Fellow
Consent	Required	Not required
Medical history	Known or accessible	Incomplete or unknown
Identification	Often known	Known, tentative, or unknown
Evidence collection	Uncommon	Routine
Photographic documentation	Inconsistent, educational	Routine
External and internal examination	Emphasis on pathology	Emphasis on TOD/PMI, injuries, and pathology
Postmortem testing	Superior sample quality Limitation in clinical lab testing on postmortem samples Emphasis on documentation of infection	Sample quality variable Designated instrumentation for postmortem testing Emphasis on documentation of intoxicants
Reporting	PAD, FAD, clinicopathologic summary Not public record	Final official report, verdict, opinion summary, ancillary reports Some reports public record

References

1. Shojania KG, Burton EC, McDonald KM, Goldman L. Changes in rates of autopsy-detected diagnostic errors over time: A systematic review. *JAMA*. 2003;289(21):2849-56.

2. Burton EC. The autopsy: A professional responsibility in assuring quality of care. *Am J Med Qual.* 2002;17(2):56-60.

3. Frohlich S, Ryan O, Murphy N, et.al. Discrepancies between clinical and autopsy diagnosis in liver transplant recipients-a case series. *Acta Gastroenterol Belg.* 2013;76(4):429-32.

4. Burton, EC, Collins KA. Autopsy rate and physician attitudes toward autopsy. Available at: www.emedicine.medscape.com/article/1705948-overview . Accessed 2/4/2016.

5. Geller, SA. Who will do my autopsy? *Arch Pathol Lab Med.*2015;139(5):578-80.

6. Hoyert DL. The changing profile of autopsied deaths in the United States, 1972-2007. NCHS Data Brief #67, Aug. 2011. Available at: www.cdc.gov/nchs/data/databriefs/db67.pdf. Accessed 2/6/2016.

7. Joint Commission on Accreditation of Healthcare Organizations. (January 1, 2004). Crosswalk of 2003 Medical Staff Standards for Hospitals to 2004 Medical Staff Standards for Hospitals. Available at: www.jointcommission.org/accreditation/hospitals.aspx. Accessed 3/13/2016.

8. American Society for Clinical Pathology. Policy Statement-Autopsy (Policy Number 91-01). 2005. Available at: www.ascp.org/pdf/Autopsy.aspx. Accessed 3/13/2016.

9. Shojania KG and Burton EC. The vanishing nonforensic autopsy. *N Engl. J Med.* 2008;358(9):873-75.

10. Jauhar, S. Bring Back the Autopsy. The New York Times. March 3, 2016. Available at: www.nytimes.com/2016/03/03/opinion/bring-back-the-autopsy.html?rref=collection%2Fcolumn%2Fsandeep-jauhar&action&_r=0 . Accessed 3/20/2016.

11. Occupational Health and Safety Administration: Bloodborne Pathogen Fact Sheet. Available at: www.osha.gov/OshDoc/data_BloodborneFacts/bbfact03.pdf . Accessed 3/6/2016.

12. Laboratory Biosafety Level Criteria. Centers for Disease Control and Prevention. Available at: www.cdc.gov/biosafety/publications/bmbl5/BMBL5_sect_IV.pdf. Accessed 3/6/2016.

13. Hutchins GM, Berman JJ, Moore W, Hanzlick R, and the Autopsy Committee of the College of American Pathologists. Practice Guidelines for Autopsy Pathology-autopsy reporting. *Arch Pathol Lab Med.* 1999;123(11):1085-92.

14. National Association of Medical Examiners. Forensic Autopsy Performance Standards. Available at: www.mtf.org/pdf/name_standards_2006.pdf. Accessed 5/22/2016.

15. Autopsy: Aiding the Living By Understanding Death. 2001. College of American Pathologists. Available at: www.cap.org . Accessed 3/20/2016.

16. Sample autopsy consent form. College of American Pathologists. Available at:www.cap.org/apps/docs/committees/autopsy/sample_autopsy_consent form.pdf . Accessed 11/12/2016. Accessed 3/20/2016.

17. Bhalia A. Bedside point of care toxicology screens in the ED: Utility and pitfalls. *Int J Crit Illn Inj Sci*. 2014;4(3):257-60.

18. Tenore PL. Advanced urine toxicology testing. *J Addict Dis.* 2010;29(4):436-48.

19. Armstrong EJ, Jenkins AJ, Sebrosky GF, Balraj EK. An unsusual fatality in a child due to oxycodone. *Am J Forensic Med Pathol.* 2004;25(4):338-41.

20. Armstrong EJ, Engelhart DA, Jenkins AJ, Balraj EK. Homicidal ethylene glycol intoxication: A report of a case. *Am J Forensic Med Pathol.* 2006; 27(2):151-55.

21. Tang MH et. al. Two cases of severe intoxication associated with analytically confirmed use of the novel psychoactive substances 25B-NBOMe and 25C-NBOMe. *Clin Toxicol (Phila)*. 2014;52(5):561-65.

22. Hanzlick RL. A synoptic review of the 1954 "Model Postmortem Examinations Act". *Acad Forensic Pathol.* 2014;4(4):451-54.

23. Peterson GF, Clark SC. Forensic autopsy performance standards. National Association of Medical Examiners; October 16, 2006:4. Available at: www.mtf.org/pdf/name_standards_2006.pdf. Accessed 9/5/2016.

24. Centers for Disease Control and Prevention. Public Health Law Program. Does state law mandate that autopsies be performed by pathologists? Available at: www.cdc.gov/phlp/publications/coroner/autopsy.html. Accessed 7/3/2016.

25. Dolinak D, Guilevardo J. Automatic implantable cardioverter defibrillator rhythm strip data as used in interpretation of a motor vehicle accident. *Am J Forensic Med Pathol.* 2001;22(3):256-60.

CHAPTER 6

FORENSIC PATHOLOGY

Introduction

The modern definition of **forensic science** is the application of scientific methods and techniques to the investigation of crime and is heavily rooted in biology, chemistry, and physics. More broadly, forensic science encompasses many of the specialized disciplines that have already been referenced in previous chapters. **Forensic pathology** is a subspecialty of pathology and a practice of medicine. It specifically involves the application of medicine to the resolution of legal and criminal matters and also falls under the umbrella of forensic science. Of equal importance are the complementary and supportive roles that forensic pathology practice plays in the practice of clinical medicine. The autopsy and the microscope are the main tools utilized by the practitioner, the forensic pathologist, "the family physician to the bereaved" [1] and the voice of the departed.

The origin of the application of the autopsy to the resolution of legal matters dates back hundreds of years and spans continents and cultural revolutions [2]. In the United States, forensic pathology formally became a subspecialty in 1959 with the first group of pathologists to complete the formalized period of fellowship training [3]. The practice had been applied on a governmental level nearly 300 years previous to that time, however [2]. As part of concentrated efforts towards the development and evolution of forensic pathology as a subspecialty practice of medicine, numerous textbooks have been published including Adelson's *The Pathology of Homicide*, Knight's *Forensic Pathology*, Spitz and Fisher's *Medicolegal Investigation of Death*, Simpson's *Forensic Medicine*, Dolinak's *Forensic Pathology-Principles and Practice*, and *Forensic Pathology* by Drs. Dominick and Vincent DiMaio. This is but a short list of the vast number of books in which the authors have combined the fruits of their own research and practice experience with the contributions of innumerable forensic science and forensic medicine professionals.

The evolution of the practice of forensic pathology continues and its momentum will depend on the continued recognition of its vital role in the practice of medicine, public health education, and the carriage of justice.

6.1 Forensic Pathology Training

Anatomic and clinical pathology (AP and CP) comprise the 2 major divisions of pathology under which fall multiple subspecialties: blood banking/transfusion medicine, chemical pathology, clinical informatics, dermatopathology, hematopathology, medical microbiology, molecular genetic pathology, neuropathology, pediatric pathology, and forensic pathology. A foundation in anatomic pathology, which currently requires 3 years of training, is necessary prior to subsequent training in forensic pathology. Alternatively, one may choose the AP/CP track, which adds an additional year of training.

Ideally, the first introduction to forensic pathology is didactic instruction preceding or following a 2-4-week rotation at the local medical examiner's or coroner's office where additional instruction is provided, all of which facilitate preparation for the pertinent part of the resident in-service examination (RISE). During the rotation period, the pathology resident is provided exposure to components and concepts of medicolegal death investigation including scene/history analysis, the forensic autopsy, postmortem toxicology and chemistry, forensic scientific techniques, and death certification. Observation of court proceedings and expert testimony given by a forensic pathologist may also be afforded to the rotating resident. Optimally, this initial introduction is scheduled to occur during the first year of residency which allows the resident time to further develop any interest by scheduling additional elective time and establishing mentorship with a practicing forensic pathologist in order to strengthen his or her candidacy for a fellowship position.

The pathology resident who has successfully completed anatomic (or anatomic and clinical) pathology residency training in a program accredited by the Accreditation Council for Graduate Medical Education (ACGME) or its international equivalent, has become qualified to sit for or has taken and passed the AP or AP/CP board examination as approved by the American Board of Pathology (ABP), and has cultivated an interest in forensic pathology, will proceed to secure fellowship training in forensic pathology for a period of 1 year. During that time, the Fellow will receive supervised training and gain practical experience in all aspects of medicolegal death investigation, forensic autopsy performance, expert medical testimony and cause and manner-of-death determination with death certification. Professional development through teaching and scholarly research and publication are supported and/or strongly encouraged. This comprehensive training in an ACGME-accredited program will well position the fellow for success on the board examination and for competent practice as a board certified forensic pathologist. The total time of postgraduate training invested is 4 years for the AP/FP track and 5 years for the AP/CP/FP track rivaling or surpassing the required years of training of other specialties and subspecialties in clinical medicine.

6.2 The Current Crisis of the Supply of Forensic Pathologists in the United States

Currently, a critical deficit in the number of practicing board certified forensic pathologists (BC-FPs) exists in the United States. Based on the geographical distribution and needs of the population, it has been estimated that between 1,100 and 1,200 BC-FPs are required to conduct forensic autopsies, however; only approximately 500 forensic pathologists are currently practicing full-time [4,5,6]. Furthermore, the yearly number of FP fellows that complete fellowship training, become board certified, and enter practice has been too low (latest figure of 21) and it is projected to take 25 years to attain the needed numbers of practicing FPs based on current population numbers and the low numbers of trained FPs entering practice [4,5,6]. There are many reasons leading up to this critical shortage including importantly:

- Under-recruitment of medical students into pathology
- Lack of inclusion of introductory forensic pathology lectures in medical school curricula
- Lack of availability of elective rotations in forensic pathology for medical students in some locales
- Rotation in forensic pathology by pathology residents beyond the first year of training
- High student debt, low compensation of FPs, and lack of federally funded student loan forgiveness programs for government-employed FPs

The remedies for most of these problems may seem obvious but the implementation of them would require reversal of current practices. Exposure to gross anatomy and microanatomy is being increasingly reduced to virtual/electronic learning platforms in many medical schools. Fewer students are provided donor cadavers as their primary anatomic learning tool and fewer of them learn how to use a microscope to examine histologically prepared tissues.

During the first and second years of medical school, students should receive 1-2-hour blocks of introductory forensic pathology instruction as part of the series of basic pathology lectures. Material on the pathophysiological processes with lethal potential inclusive of trauma sequela should be presented and will facilitate the introduction and comprehension of the concepts of cause and manner of death. At this time, students should also be required to view a forensic autopsy as a way to introduce the concept of clinicopathologic correlation. The early years of medical school education is the optimal time to pique interest in the field of pathology including forensic pathology and to prompt selection of pathology rotations in the third and fourth years or a post-sophomore pathology fellowship. During the third and fourth years, students should elect to spend 2 to 4 weeks at a medical examiner's or coroner's office to gain additional exposure to gross anatomy through autopsy observation while learning to recognize external and internal signs of disease and injury. During such elective time, the student should also learn which deaths are reportable to the ME/C and how to properly formulate the cause and manner of death on a death certificate. In many locales, forensic pathologists donate considerable amounts of valuable time on a routine basis to instruct medical students regarding medicolegal death investigation. Ideally, medical schools should reciprocate and establish an official memorandum of understanding that includes not only academic appointment but also provides stipends for the services of these dedicated professionals. Currently, the Cuyahoga County Medical Examiner's Office (CCMEO) in Cleveland, Ohio offers a 2-4 week comprehensive elective rotation in forensic pathology to medical, osteopathic, and physician assistant students. Autopsy demonstration classes are also currently offered.

It is the opinion of the author, as a result of personal and observational experience, that forensic pathology is not always perceived as a viable career option by hospital-based attending pathologists and pathology residency program directors. It is also acknowledged that pathology residency programs have fewer residents to handle service work and any time that the resident spends away from service shifts the workload onto others. Because of perceptions and workload constraints, often the resident's first exposure to forensic pathology is not until the third or fourth year of residency and he/she may or may not have received basic didactic lectures. By that time, whether on an AP-only or AP/CP track, many residents have already decided upon a subspecialty and have interviewed and signed on with a fellowship program and otherwise have little interest in forensic pathology. Others may have considered forensic pathology as a viable career option had earlier exposure during the first year of residency been afforded to them. Currently, CCMEO accommodates pathology residents from 3 local teaching hospitals for 2 weeks of comprehensive medicolegal death investigation introduction, with first-year residents coming from 2 of the 3 hospitals. Didactic lectures given by the staff forensic pathologists are also provided to all pathology residents on an as-needed basis. While the pathology programs from these local hospitals require 2 weeks of exposure, other programs across the country require an entire month, but not necessarily during the first year of training.

High job satisfaction, low burnout potential, financial security, and work-life balance are top determining factors in the choice of a practice specialty and subspecialty in light of burdensome debt incurred during the years as an undergraduate and/or medical student. Compensation of a practicing forensic pathologist (either as a deputy ME or deputy C), who is often based in a government-operated ME/C's office, averages approximately $185,000/year with *chief* medical examiners and *deputy chief* medical examiners compensated on average $220,000/year and $190,000/year, respectively [7]. The yearly compensation amount for full-time hospital pathologists is approximately $335,000 [8]. Other clinical specialties and subspecialties have much higher yearly compensation packages than forensic pathology as well. The choice becomes clear when considering the low pay, the physical and mental demands, and the unpredictability of death encountered in forensic pathology practice, even in light of more regular work hours and regular on-call scheduling. All of these factors combine into a major impediment to increasing the supply of FPs and ameliorating the crisis which will continue to accelerate as currently practicing FPs retire, change careers, or die. National scientific commissions and working groups, chief medical examiners and coroners, televised documentaries, journal articles, and news reports have in the recent years put the crisis at the forefront of the minds of the public and the politicians. The politicians working at both the local and federal levels are instrumental in helping to secure funding for medical examiner/coroner (ME/C) offices that can be used in part to increase compensation and attract well qualified candidates [4,9,10].

Despite the current challenges facing the practice of forensic pathology, FPs have the amazing ability to cope with and surmount the demands of practice which is greatly aided by the camaraderie and exchange of ideas with colleagues within the workplace, at yearly national meetings, and on electronic platforms such as listservs. They experience a great degree of satisfaction not only from these professional interactions but also from interaction with the medical, legal, and scientific communities, and importantly the bereaved families, providing them with answers and understanding.

6.3 The Forensic Pathologist's Role in Quality Assurance and Improvement of Patient Care and Public Health

On many levels, forensic pathologists are an integral part in the delivery of health care and are monitors of public health and safety. The autopsy report and death certificate are just two of many mediums with which important circumstantial, medical, and cause-of-death information is disseminated to the clinicians, families, and the public. Detailed descriptions of injuries found in forensic autopsy reports are used clinically for the calculation of the Injury Severity Scale (ISS) and the Abbreviated Injury Scale (AIS) which in turn are used to optimize management of trauma patients [11]. Death scene, autopsy, and laboratory reports are all generated by ME/C offices and these reports contain detailed information about hazardous environments, chronic medical conditions, infectious disease, therapeutic interventions/devices and illicit drug and medication usage that are reviewed and interpreted by forensic pathologists. Many ME/C offices publish statistical data not only regarding the various causes and manners of death, but also regarding geographical features, demographical features, and temporal associations. Local monitoring of death trends associated with clandestinely manufactured drugs of abuse and periodic notification of the public directly inform and assist in the mobilization of the law makers, police, and medical professionals towards action and prevention [12]. Aside from statistical, report-based data, retained tissue and fluid samples routinely collected during a medicolegal autopsy may be useful in public health studies regarding certain age-associated medical conditions.

As a kind community health provider, forensic pathologists working in ME/C offices provide expertise via participation at hospital trauma conferences, morbidity and mortality conferences, domestic violence death review committees, and child death review committees, to name a few. These focus groups comprise of not only forensic pathologists but also clinicians, law enforcement officers, social workers, and legal professionals. These groups work collaboratively providing a multidisciplinary approach to identifying risk factors and ways to prevent or reduce future morbidity, mortality, and risky behavior. Some level of grief counseling may also be provided by the forensic pathologist or wholly by mental health professionals working in or affiliated with ME/C offices.

Clinicians should take advantage of any opportunity their local ME/C's office may offer to gain a fundamental understanding of medicolegal death investigation and the interface it has with clinical practice. Residents in the primary care specialties including emergency medicine, internal medicine, family medicine, obstetrics/gynecology, surgery, and psychiatry would especially benefit. Attending physicians, physician assistants, and nurses also practicing in those same primary care specialties would also benefit greatly. Aside from attendance to morbidity and mortality conferences, requiring trainees to visit the local ME/C's office in order to observe triage of jurisdictional cases, observe workup of a sudden death by way of autopsy, and receive customized instruction on death certification would enrich the training experience. Department heads or chief residents in the primary care specialties and on the oncology and hospice services should solicit lectures for staff members on reportable deaths and death certification from the local ME/C or health department. Moreover, a formal memorandum of understanding between residency training programs in the primary care specialties and the local medical examiner or coroner's office should be established along with academic appointment and provision of stipends for the forensic pathology staff involved in the education of their residents.

6.4 Applications in Forensic Pathology in the Workup of Jurisdictional Deaths

Deaths accepted under the jurisdiction of the ME/C are further reviewed on a near daily basis. These are sudden, unexpected, unexplained, unnatural, and unattended deaths as required by state law. As a most recent perspective, in

2004, approximately 30-40% or 1 million deaths occurring in the United States were referred to ME/C offices with jurisdiction taken over approximately 50%, or 500,000 those [13]. Not all jurisdictional deaths will need determination of the cause and manner of death with performance of an autopsy, an important point for morgue attendants and clinicians to convey to families when the patient has expired in a medical facility. Furthermore, all jurisdictional deaths will have the death certificate completed by the ME/C or forensic pathologist, whether or not an autopsy is performed.

The decision to perform an autopsy is made on a case-by-case basis, within the context of the history and circumstances surrounding the death and increasingly, based on the adequacy of staffing and resources of a given office. *To reiterate, an autopsy will not be performed on every medical examiner's or coroner's case.* In some offices, an external examination of the body with sampling of bodily fluids for laboratory storage or testing will be performed. Results of any testing along with review of pertinent records will ensue with subsequent determination of the cause and manner of death and certification of the same. In other offices and in certain cases, the cause of death will be determined by review of pertinent records only in absence of an external examination (or viewing of the body) and sampling of bodily fluids.

Deaths resulting from the acute or delayed effects of known or suspected homicidal violence or resulting from the acute effects of suicidal injury or overdose should be verified with an autopsy as it is of utmost importance to document distinguishing features of these two types of deaths with correlation with the historical information as there could be very different investigative and legal ramifications if misidentified. Delayed deaths due to complications stemming from homicidal violence should be autopsied as it is important document the temporal association between the initial injury and any ensuing complications and to evaluate the significance of any pre-existing and co-existing conditions. An autopsy may not be performed in every case of suicide if, for example, there was a prolonged in-hospital survival interval or when family requests that no autopsy be performed *and* the history of the events leading to hospitalization have been documented and can be verified to be suicidal in nature. Inter- and *intra*-office variability, regarding autopsy performance will apply to other types of cases. For example, not every office will perform an autopsy on every accidental death such as those resulting from drug overdoses or motor vehicle collisions.

Sudden and unexpected deaths of likely natural causes but with inadequate history in persons 60 years of age or less often need determination of the cause of death with the aid of an autopsy, with cardiovascular disease commonly found in the 40-60-year age range. Chronic alcoholics with evidence of terminal active alcohol use may die of natural disease sequelae related to alcohol use but they are also prone to injury from falls and assaults. The autopsy and postmortem testing will document the extent of acute and chronic alcohol-associated disease and any injury for the most accurate cause and manner-of-death determination. If warranted, toxicological and chemistry testing will be performed even when an autopsy is not needed such as in the postmortem diagnosis of diabetic ketoacidosis in an older person with otherwise well-documented natural disease and no significant interval injury. Overall, the forensic pathologist must recognize the diseases that have lethal potential amongst any incidental findings discovered at autopsy and know that some will be grossly or microscopically evident and others will not.

Forensic pathologists are trained specifically to recognize and assess not only disease conditions but also injury and to determine whether the cause of death is due to disease alone, injury alone, or as a result of a combination of the two. Though seemingly straightforward, these determinations may be difficult owing to long intervals of time that may have transpired between the injury and death or between the onset of the disease and death and requires application of not only knowledge of forensic pathology but also of general medicine. Moreover, some natural disease or therapy-related manifestations mimic those associated with impact injury such as bruising in coagulopathic patients with chronic liver disease or subdural hemorrhage in patients treated with anti-coagulant or anti-platelet medications. The development of any interval complications stemming from the disease or injury or the occurrence of intervening disease or injury not associated with the original injury must also be evaluated. With any contribution of injury to the death (i.e. injury linked to decline in baseline health status), even in the setting of significant natural disease, the manner of death is then not purely natural. It must then be determined whether the injury happened by **accident**, was due to self-harm (**suicide**), or was as a result of the willful action or inaction of another (**homicide**). These classifications of death are collectively known as **manner of death**. When injury (and any complication thereof) played a part in the death and the circumstances or the situation in which it arose (or the manner) cannot be determined, then the **undetermined** classification is applied. It must be clarified that in forensic pathology practice, *injury* refers not only to physical trauma but also encompasses less visually obvious changes such as those resulting from intoxication/poisoning or asphyxia. Thus, there are a total of 5 classifications of manner of death used by FPs: natural, accident, suicide, homicide, and undetermined.

Over a career time, a forensic pathologist encounters thousands of natural and non-natural types of deaths spanning all age groups. Natural deaths are the most common type of deaths encountered accounting for between 40-50% of deaths received in ME/C offices with cardiovascular disease occupying the number one position, followed by respiratory and central nervous system diseases as reflected in the Nation's health statistics. Table 6.1 lists some commonly encountered natural disease entities as listed on death certificates. In order of frequency by manner-of-death classification, natural deaths are followed by accidental, suicidal, homicidal, and undetermined types (or manners). Examples of accidental deaths include falls with craniocerebral injury, illicit and prescription drug overdoses, asphyxia by choking on food, and deaths from motor vehicle collisions. Examples of common types of suicidal deaths include deaths due to gunshot wounds, overdoses, and asphyxial hanging. Examples of common types of homicidal deaths include deaths due to gunshot wounds, blunt force trauma, stab wounds, and strangulation.

Deaths unique to infants and children include those due to motor vehicle accidents, drownings, physical abuse and neglect, medical neglect, and congenital and acquired disease and must be carefully evaluated. Infant deaths associated with unsafe sleep arrangement such as bed-sharing or hazardous bedding may be designated as a **Sudden Unexplained Infant Death (SUID)** after a thorough review of the medical history, investigative information and autopsy results that lack diagnostic information. In sudden infant deaths lacking hazardous sleep conditions and with negative investigative and non-diagnostic autopsy-related findings, the designation of **Sudden Infant Death Syndrome (SIDS)**, a subcategory of SUID, may be in order. Sudden deaths associated with a history of unexplained respiratory ailments or skeletal injury may represent abuse from smothering or inflicted trauma which will require autopsy performance with histological and radiological study, performance of toxicology and chemistry testing, and careful review of medical records. This is necessary in order to document the acuity or chronicity of bona fide inflicted injury or provide an alternate explanation through diagnosis of natural disease co-existing with inconsequential injury. For example, it must be determined whether a sudden death of a toddler with multiple fractures of the axial and/or appendicular skeleton represents inflicted injury versus some type of genetic disorder of collagen synthesis or a nutritional deficiency. A high degree of medical certainty is necessary when the determination of inflicted injury is made as the FP must communicate his/her findings to law enforcement which will initiate or prompt continuation of an investigation as to how the injuries came to be and who caused them. Sudden death in children with non-diagnostic gross and microscopic pathological findings may warrant further testing including testing for inborn errors of metabolism and cardiac genetic defects. Historical reports of any prior involvement of caregivers with child protection services are another important source of information in the workup of child deaths. Locally and state-based child death review teams systematically collect social, medical, and cause-of-death-data in order to identify risk factors and patterns in infant/child deaths in an effort to prevent future deaths through national publication of recommendations [14]. Forensic pathologists are an integral part of this multidisciplinary team.

Like infants and children, the elderly represent a more vulnerable group in our society. Unlike infants and children however, they more often have chronic natural disease of one or more organ systems that can lead to death whether suddenly or expectedly. Clinically, sudden deaths in the elderly are more likely to be attributed to natural disease, especially if already documented in the medical record. Debility from chronic natural diseases such as cardiovascular and cerebrovascular diseases, diabetes, and periodontal disease with tooth loss may also precipitate accidental types of death such as death from choking. The presumption of cardiovascular disease as a proximate cause of cardiopulmonary arrest or rapid deterioration may preclude prompt clinical diagnosis of choking leading to preventable morbidity and mortality [15]. Due to the frailty and vulnerability, whether as a result of progressive neurodegenerative disease or immobility by other chronic diseases, our elders may suffer untoward death by physical abuse or neglect. Manifestations of physical abuse and neglect overlap those of natural disease and aging changes and the important task of the forensic pathologist when evaluating deaths under these circumstances is to decipher the difference by way of competent autopsy performance with postmortem testing, careful review of medical records and if necessary, request investigation by law enforcement [16]. Multidisciplinary elder death review teams work locally with medical examiners and coroners to investigate elder deaths suspected to involve abuse, neglect, and exploitation with contribution from social workers, clinicians, attorneys, long-term care professionals, and financial institutions [17].

Aside from accidents, homicides, and suicides, FPs are often involved in the workup of sudden and unexpected deaths that occur during hospitalization and treatment for natural disease and injury or those that occur following discharge. These include deaths stemming from misdiagnosis, delayed diagnosis, partial diagnosis, and non-diagnosis. Any legal inquiry pursuant to malpractice claims that may follow will require the expertise provided by the forensic pathologist whether during pre-trial meetings, at deposition, or during live court proceedings [18,19,20]. Examples of such deaths include illicit drug and prescription overdoses, pulmonary arterial embolism following initiation of oral contraceptives, fat/bone marrow embolism following long bone fracture with surgical intervention, acute myocardial infarct with atypical clinical presentation, atypical presentation of ruptured aortic aneurysm, café coronary (asphyxia by choking on food), vascular perforation after catheter placement, vascular perforation during disc surgery, iatrogenic perforation of viscera during placement of tubes and catheters, cardiac arrest following administration of incorrect medication, and metabolic complications due to failure to restart medications following surgery. Other types of deaths are those that occur during or following surgical and non-surgical therapeutic interventions for natural disease, such as a death occurring after perforation of the aorta during lumbar disc surgery or after administration of thrombolytic medication for ischemic stroke. In some jurisdictions, the latter type of death is referred to as a **therapeutic complication** and the manner of death will be classified as such. Further discussion regarding deaths associated with therapy and surgery is presented in Chapter 8, section 8.5.

This section presents but a few of numerous examples published and unpublished alike, of applied forensic pathology. Furthermore, the forensic autopsy and postmortem testing provide the gold standard means by which to determine not only the cause and manner of death but also to provide a quality assurance measure through confirmation of clinicopathologic correlation or to illuminate incongruences between cause-of-death findings and clinical workup.

6.5 Injury Types: A Primer for Clinical Practitioners

Forensic pathologists identify and interpret injuries regularly. The type, size, distribution, acuteness or healing stage of both external and internal injury often provide clues regarding the death circumstances if not the cause of death altogether. It is important that clinicians and clinical trainees correctly identify external injuries and to document them using the correct terminology in the medical record that may be subsequently read and interpreted by others, including third party medical, legal, and insurance professionals. Clinicians who practice in the primary care specialties may at some point during their career encounter or treat injuries sustained by victims of assault and the accurate description of these injuries will facilitate any police investigation into the circumstances surrounding the assault inclusive of the type of weapon used on the victim. Not surprisingly, surgical and emergency medicine physicians, physician assistants, and nurses are far more adept at injury recognition and description as a direct result of their training and practice experience. Unfortunately, the physical examination of the skin is either overlooked altogether or more often cursory with description of only the hue, tactile temperature, and degree of moistness. Frequently omitted are descriptive details of injury and scars, especially surgical scars. The following general overview of cutaneous injury types will provide the clinical practitioner with a good working knowledge applicable to the physical examination of the patient. The overview is not meant to be an all-inclusive description of the many variations. Illustrative images of select injuries appear near the end of this chapter.

6.5.1 Blunt Force Injury

Blunt force injury (alternatively-blunt force trauma or blunt impact injury) is the most common type of injury encountered in forensic cases and is more often an incidental finding and not part of the cause of death. It is the result of a number of different incidents including normal activities of daily living, falls, transportation-related accidents, assaults, and industrial accidents, sometimes with a pre-death survival interval and corresponding evidence of healing. Often, this type of injury is sustained upon terminal collapse resulting in injury commonly of the head and extremities, the extent of which may or may not be sufficient to constitute a cause or contributing factor in the death.

Blunt force injury is the result of the transfer of kinetic energy from an object or a surface to some part of the body. This happens either by direct impact to the body by a blunt object (including by an extremity of an assailant) or as a result of a part of the body impacting a non-sharp surface. Sudden deceleration of a body in motion with terminal impact onto a surface can cause not only cutaneous injury at the point of impact but also internal injury to mobile regional anatomic structures. As an example, the more mobile proximal descending aorta (relative to the proximal ascending aorta tethered at the level of the ligamentum arteriosum) can become partially or totally avulsed as a result of shearing forces precipitated by sudden deceleration of the body as can occur in motor vehicle collisions. Moreover, significant internal injury resulting from deceleration-type forces can occur in the absence of significant cutaneous injury.

With direct impact, the characteristics of the object, the velocity and force of the impact, the location and surface area of the body affected, and the integrity of the skin are important factors that determine the extent and severity of injury caused by the striking object. Sometimes, blunt impacts cause little or no external injury but significant internal injury, due in part to the rapid absorption and dissipation of kinetic energy and the thickness and elasticity of the impacted body region. The scalp and the abdominal wall are representative of such body regions whereby the inherent shock absorptive characteristics added with the presence of body hair and/or clothing in some cases attenuate injury to the cutaneous layer. Furthermore, head impacts can cause subdural hemorrhage without visible scalp injury and abdominal impacts can cause extensive visceral laceration or intestinal injury but without visible abdominal bruising. In infants, children, and even the elderly, multiple blunt force injuries in various stages of healing, on atypical body regions, or that are otherwise inconsistent with the explanation provided by caregivers or inconsistent with the developmental stage and degree of mobility, should serve as red-flags to clinicians for possible abuse. Clinical practitioners by law are mandated reporters of any suspected physical abuse.

The dissipation of the kinetic energy resulting from impact may be significant enough to cause one or a combination of 4 general types of blunt force injury:

- **Abrasion**: impact or friction causing disruption of the epidermis, dermis, or mucosal surface; ex. scrapes or skinning
- **Contusion**: impact causing disruption of blood vessels with localized extravasation of blood and non-blanchable discoloration; ex. bruise
- **Laceration**: impact causing irregular tearing or crushing leaving bridging of blood vessels and connective tissue; ex. tear

- **Fracture**: impact causing breach of tensile force of bone or cartilage with or without partial or complete separation, dislocation, or injury to surrounding or adjacent tissues

The differentiating features of cutaneous blunt force injury are usually easily discernible. Abrasions feel rough whereas contusions feel smooth owing to the intactness of the epidermis. Abrasions may also bleed if dermal and subcutaneous blood vessels are involved imparting a brown or red color before healing with eschar formation. Lacerations are often misidentified as cuts or stab wounds which are sharp force injuries. Like cuts and stab wounds, the wound edges of lacerations at times look smooth and regular, but more often they are irregular. Classically, the presence of **tissue bridging** distinguishes lacerations. An impact may produce injury comprised of more than one type such as an abraded laceration, abraded laceration with contusion, abraded contusion, lacerated contusion, or an open fracture where the displaced fractured end lacerates and the overlying skin. Although not externally apparent, contusion and laceration of viscera is also observed such as with pulmonary contusion from direct impact, pulmonary laceration from displaced rib fractures, and hepatic or splenic laceration from direct impact or compressive forces.

Depending on the characteristics of the impacting object, the type of surface impacted by the body, or the way in which the body impacts a surface, abrasions can be further categorized into subtypes:

- **Linear**: produced by a narrow or pointy object; ex. scratch
- **Broad**: movement of body along broad surface; ex. road rash
- **Patterned**: takes on the shape of the object; ex. gravel abrasions from impact with pavement, 'tram track' abrasions from impacts with elongated objects (i.e. whips, pipes and boards), bitemarks, seat belt shoulder harness, therapeutic devices
- **Stretch**: overstretching of skin, especially flexion points of extremities
- **Impact**: perpendicular forces; ex. impact with hammer
- **Graze**: glancing forces; ex. bullet graze wound

In the living, contusions resolve over time changing color as the heme component of hemoglobin is enzymatically broken down into biliverdin and bilirubin and thus the change in appearance from red/blue/purple (acute) to green/brown/yellow (resolving). The time line for resolution of contusions exhibits inter- and intra-individual variability and also depends on size and depth of injury. The same contusion can have a variegated appearance representing acute and resolving changes. Like abrasions, contusions can have a patterned appearance, taking on the shape of the impacting or impacted object or surface. **Ecchymosis** is a term often used interchangeably with contusion as the definition and appearance of each are similar. Unlike contusion, an ecchymosis may or may not result from trauma and it is associated with senile skin changes, coagulopathy, venipunctures, and an underlying or adjacent fracture. Ecchymosis of certain body regions can be an indication of significant underlying injury such as **periorbital ecchymosis** (anterior cranial fossa or nasal fracture) and **mastoid ecchymosis** (**Battle's sign**, middle cranial fossa fracture). Periorbital and mastoid ecchymosis are not sites of impact and instead are a result of impact injury to nearby cranial skeletal anatomy accompanied by hemorrhage extending from the fracture site and tracking along subcutaneous tissue planes. **Petechial hemorrhage** is seen on skin and visceral surfaces and is the result of a number of non-mechanical and mechanical causes. These include consumptive coagulopathy associated with infections, resuscitative chest compressions, constricting therapeutic devices like blood pressure cuffs, positional and mechanical asphyxia, and compression of the neck vessels in ligature and manual strangulation.

6.5.2 Sharp Force Injury

Sharp force injury is caused by sharp-edged objects and surfaces leaving wounds with smooth edges *without* tissue bridging as the tissue has been severed. It is divided into 3 general types:

- **Incised**: wounds that are longer than deep; ex. a cut or slash
- **Stab**: wounds that are deeper than long
- **Chop**: caused by weighty edged instruments like axes or boat propellers; wounds may have an abraded component

The configuration of a given sharp force injury can provide information as to what caused it. Examples include paired triangular wounds (open scissors), paired round puncture wounds (barbecue fork), single puncture wound (icepick or screwdriver), jagged irregular wounds (glass shards), and short single or crisscross incised wounds or dicing injury (from shattered tempered glass). Single-edged knives may produce wounds with blunting at one end of the wound. Wounds produced by doubled-edged knives may lack blunting of both ends. Wounds produced by either types inserted up to the handle often produce wounds with blunting at both ends in addition to abrasion or contusion from impact of the handle or the assailant's hand gripped around the handle. Serrated knives drawn across the skin at an acute angle may leave regularly-spaced parallel linear abrasions corresponding to the serrated edge.

It is preferable that stab wounds and other penetrating wounds not be used as ports for tube or catheter insertion or as starting points for surgical incisions if at all possible, with the understanding that the patient's condition may be critical and the need for emergent procedures becomes priority. If it is necessary to utilize these injuries as ports and the patient subsequently expires, then this should be documented in the medical record and directly communicated to the forensic pathologist performing the autopsy. Surgical incisions such as incisions for chest tube placement can have the appearance of or be interpreted as stab wounds especially if there is perforation of the underlying lung which is also a known complication of chest tube placement. Thus, it is preferable that chest tubes be left in place if the patient expires and becomes a ME/C's case.

6.5.3 Firearm Injuries

An injury caused by a bullet commonly fired from handguns has defining features relative to the point of entry or exit, and the resulting wound is referred to as a **gunshot wound (GSW)**. Typically, an **entrance wound** is a ¼ to ½ inch round to ovoid full-thickness skin defect, the edges of which cannot be re-approximated as the skin has been punched out and disintegrated by the bullet. The circumferential edge of the wound is typically abraded leaving a narrow pink or brown skinless edge known as **marginal abrasion**. Contact or near contact entrance wounds over bony surfaces such as the head may be stellate representing the effects of gas and pressure forced under the skin causing multiple circumferential lacerations. The lacerations can be re-approximated leaving a round to ovoid defect, complete with marginal abrasion, typical of entrance wounds in other body locations. The bullet may not enter the body but instead may either superficially or deeply graze the skin leaving an elongated abrasion or a lacerated abrasion with tags of skin along the margins.

If the muzzle end of the firearm touched (contact), nearly touched (near contact) or was a few inches away (close range) upon discharge, then a grey-black powdery substance (burned and vaporized gunpowder) may appear around the entrance wound or within the depths of the wound. This is known as **fouling** and the material will be removed by surgical skin preparations and wound care procedures. Therefore, it is important to document the presence of fouling in the medical record. If the muzzle end of the firearm was tightly against the skin upon discharge then an abraded and/or contused outline may be left, known as a **muzzle stamp** or **muzzle imprint**. These are additional examples of patterned blunt force injury produced as the skin rapidly slaps back against the firearm as the gas pressure escapes under the skin upon discharge.

The presence of **stippling** or **powder tattooing** may be noted around entrance wounds where the firearm was at an intermediate distance (approximately 2 to 3 feet) upon discharge. These red or brown punctate abrasions are caused by impacts by gunpowder particles expelled from the end of the firearm upon firing. They cannot be wiped away but will eventually heal (with or without scarring) given time after survival of the injury. Surgical defects from suturing or stapling of the wound may mimic these, thus description of stippling in the medical record will assist in distinguishing these injuries from artifacts of surgical intervention.

The bullet may possess enough kinetic energy to exit the body typically creating a smaller and more irregular skin laceration or **exit wound**, the edges of which can be re-approximated to form a complete surface. Exit wounds may be slit-like with the appearance of an incised or stab wound but with focal tissue bridging that is often visible on close inspection. Exit wounds lack marginal abrasion, fouling, and stippling. There may be bruising or abrasion adjacent to an exit wound that was covered by tight clothing or was adjacent to a firm surface. This is referred to as a **shored exit** in which the exiting bullet causes the surrounding skin to impact the overlying surface causing contusion or abrasion of the skin adjacent to the wound. For the same reasons previously stated, exit wounds should not be used as ports for therapeutic intervention unless medically necessary.

An entrance wound caused by *shotgun* ammunition at contact or close range is a large wound, typically ¾ - 1 inch and may have fouling or stippling present and is referred to as a **shotgun wound (SGW**) Unlike handguns, shotguns are typically long-barreled, smooth-bore weapons fired from the shoulder.

Contact and close-range SGWs produce devastating often rapidly fatal injuries especially with involvement of the head and torso regions. Contact SGWs of the head often appear as large gaping defects with multiple skull fractures, scalp and facial lacerations, and partial or complete ejection of the brain. A SGW from several feet way using ammunition containing pellets (shot) may or may not have a central entrance defect produced by shotgun shell. At that distance, the shotgun shell instead may only impact and abrade the skin prior to falling away, after first opening up and releasing numerous pellets. Multiple separate wounds of entry produced by the pellets may be apparent and simulate stippling but are larger in appearance. These pellets rapidly loose kinetic energy upon impact with the skin and subjacent tissues. Retained pellets will be evident on imaging studies. Some types of shotgun ammunition contain only a single slug that is similar to the prototypical bullet and can produce entry and exit wounds similar to GSWs, especially at contact or close range.

6.5.4 Stigmata of Drug Abuse

It is the author's personal experience based on the of review of thousands of medical records that the emergency medical service and hospital medical records of patients with a known history of drug abuse often do not contain pertinent information regarding the physical examination of the skin organ. The denial of drug use by a patient can often be refuted during the clinical physical examination with detection of certain skin changes, even before receipt of the urine drug screen results. In forensic cases arriving from the hospital, it is often evident that the non-therapeutic injection of substances was suspected clinically. Intravascular catheters are often found to be placed contralateral to chronically accessed sites. Intraosseous catheters are also frequently encountered in the same setting likely because the scarred peripheral sites either could not be cannulated and infused or out of concern for the risk of iatrogenic systemic bacterial contamination. Any clinical suspicion of chronic intravenous drug use evident on skin exam should be routinely documented in the medical record.

The acute and chronic stigmata of drug abuse, particularly those involving injection of substances, are often readily seen on skin examination upon external examination during a forensic autopsy on a decedent that has arrived from the hospital. Sometimes these stigmata are not readily visible because they are camouflaged by tattoos or body hair or are located on hidden areas of the body. Moreover, the clinical practitioner may not see evidence of skin injection with use of tuberculin-type needles which leave tiny red pinpoint marks that are either imperceptible or indistinguishable from normal or inflamed hair follicles. Patients addicted to illicit substances or narcotic analgesic medications may utilize indwelling catheters such as mediports (also known as portacaths) and dialysis catheters, presenting with multiple, often scabbed, puncture marks over these sites that may escape detection by the unsuspecting examiner.

Injuries caused by repeated injection of substances like heroin or crushed and dissolved pills into superficial veins will appear as clustered pinpoint defects, multiple pinpoint defects in a linear array or scattered pinpoint defects. The defects most often appear red or purple, with or without surrounding ecchymosis and with or without crusting. Repeated injection of the same site over time often results in palpable induration due to chronic inflammation and scar tissue formation and are also known as **track marks**. The most commonly accessed locations are the antecubital fossae, dorsal hand surfaces, and forearms. Other sites accessed include the sides of the neck (superficial or jugular veins), upper arms, axillae, fingers, calves, dorsum of feet, ankles, interdigital regions, scrotum, and superficial penile veins. These puncture sites may be hidden by hair (or clothing) and deciphering them form hair follicles or even folliculitis can be challenging. Other sites of access are those strategically located within tattoos such as the convergence points of spider webs where they may be imperceptible or otherwise go unnoticed. Repeated intravenous injection using contaminated needles may lead to cutaneous and subcutaneous abscess formation with ulcerated wounds that exude pus in addition to cellulitis and necrotizing fasciitis.

Usually, after all superficial venous sites have been exhausted owing to scar formation with obstruction of the lumen, the substance will be administered subcutaneously, also known as "**skin popping**". The effects of the chronic injection of cocaine which is also sometimes mixed with levamisole will cause focal skin ulceration with scarring and hypo- or hyperpigmentation leaving multiple round to ovoid lesions or scars, ½ to ¾ inch in diameter. Injection of cocaine, heroin, and other substances that may be mixed with caustic chemicals may also induce a vasculitis that then leads to skin ulceration. Many palpable indurated chronic venous access sites are also usually evident in conjunction with skin popping, representing a transition to an alternate route of drug self-administration. Like with chronic intravenous drug administrations, repeated subcutaneous injection using contaminated needles may lead to abscess formation, ulceration, deep tissue infection, and partial or complete loss of limbs and digits.

Evidence of drug use by other routes may also be noted upon physical examination. Thermal injuries to the tips of the fingers with blistering, blackening, and hardening, occur in smokers of crack cocaine as a result of prolonged repeated contact with the hot glass pipe used for smoking the substance. Insufflation or snorting of cocaine or methamphetamine may be evident not only by the residue on or within the nares but also by the presence of a perforated nasal septum. Huffing or the repeated inhalation of volatile substances from pressurized containers such as spray paint cans or computer cleaners may leave nasal abrasions, frostbite-type skin lesions of the nose and lips, or staining of the peri-oral/nasal regions or fingers by the substance. Other secondary skin changes due to allergic reactions causing pruritic urticarial lesions leading to excoriation-type abrasions may be seen. Multiple and diffuse punctate abrasions of the face and extremities have been described in users of cocaine and methamphetamine as a manifestation of the psychological effects of drug use where the user experiences the sensation of insects crawling on the skin, known as delusions of parisitosis [21].

6.5.5 Miscellaneous Injury Types

Additional less common injury types may come to the attention of the clinician and otherwise be consistent with the circumstances that led to the clinical presentation. These are electrical, thermal, or chemical injuries. **Electrical** or **electrothermal injuries** have appearances that range from white dot-like blisters to chalky white/red/black ulcerated lesions with raise borders and blanched skin at the periphery to extensive charring seen with lightning strikes. They also can have appearances that overlap injuries cause by heat or flame. **Thermal injuries** produced by heat or flame have characteristic appearances based on the depth of the injury ranging from redness and blistering (partial to full-thickness dermal injury) to charring with injury of all skin layers, muscle and bone. Scalding-type thermal injuries that are caused by contact with steam or hot liquids in infants and children may be of concern to clinicians when the pattern and location of injury is inconsistent with the explanation provided by the caretaker(s). Other patterned thermal injuries (or scars) such as ¼ to ½ inch in diameter injuries, elongated injuries, or checkerboard-like injuries on an infant or child should raise concern for abusive type injuries caused by lit cigarettes and heated implements such as curling irons or clothing irons. **Chemical burn injuries** will have characteristic appearances based on the acidity or alkalinity of the contacting substance, the concentration of the active ingredient(s), and the duration of contact with the skin. Splash and drip patterns of skin damage may also be evident.

Table 6.1 Select Natural Disease Entities in Medicolegal Cases As Entered on Death Certificates

Atherosclerotic cardiovascular disease
Hypertensive cardiovascular disease
Atherosclerotic coronary artery disease
Coronary arterial thrombosis with acute myocardial infarct
Acute myocardial infarct with spontaneous ventricular rupture and hemopericardium
Valvular heart disease (mitral valve prolapse)
Bacterial endocarditis
Ischemic cardiomyopathy
Hypertensive cerebrovascular disease with acute intracerebral hemorrhage
Spontaneous acute rupture of abdominal aortic aneurysm
Spontaneous acute ascending aortic dissection with rupture and hemopericardium
Pulmonary arterial thromboembolism due to deep vein thrombosis
Peptic ulcer disease with spontaneous acute perforation and hemoperitoneum
Chronic asthmatic bronchitis with acute bronchial asthma
Acute bronchopneumonia due to Chronic Obstructive Pulmonary Disease (pulmonary emphysema)
Hepatic encephalopathy due to alcoholic liver disease with cirrhosis
Diabetic ketoacidosis due to Type I Diabetes Mellitus
Hyperosmolar Hyperglycemic Nonketotic Syndrome due to Type 2 Diabetes Mellitus
Spontaneous acute rupture of cerebral artery aneurysm
Sudden Unexpected Death in Epilepsy
Sudden cardiac death due to obesity-associated cardiomyopathy

Figure 6.1 Patterned contusions and abrasions caused by mechanical chest compression device

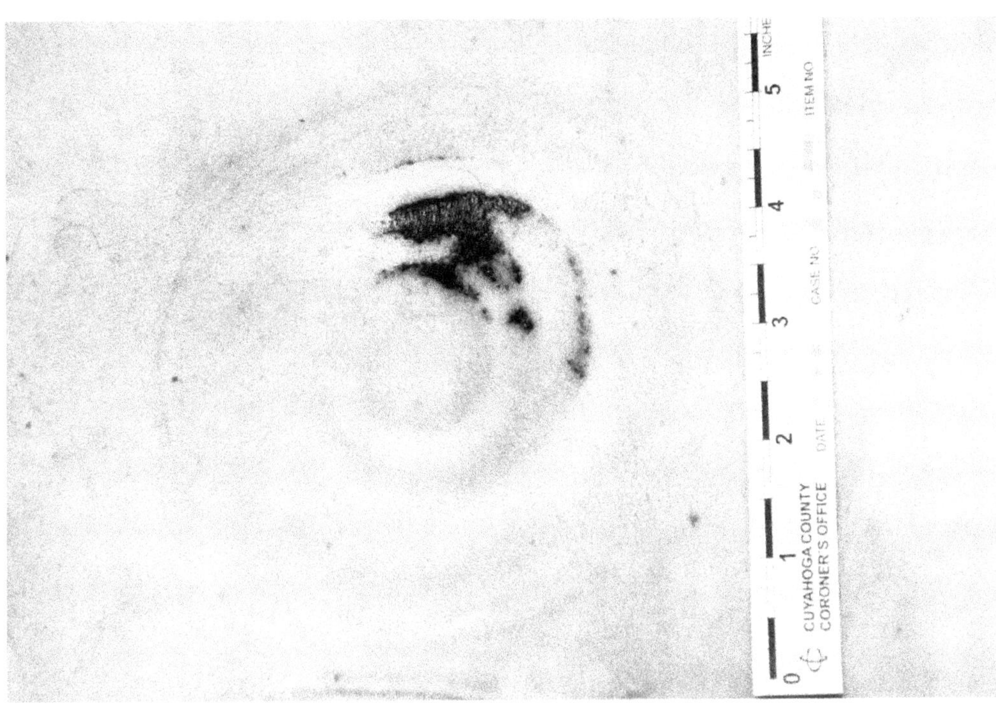

Figure 6.2 Shoulder harness abrasion of driver, victim of motor vehicle collision

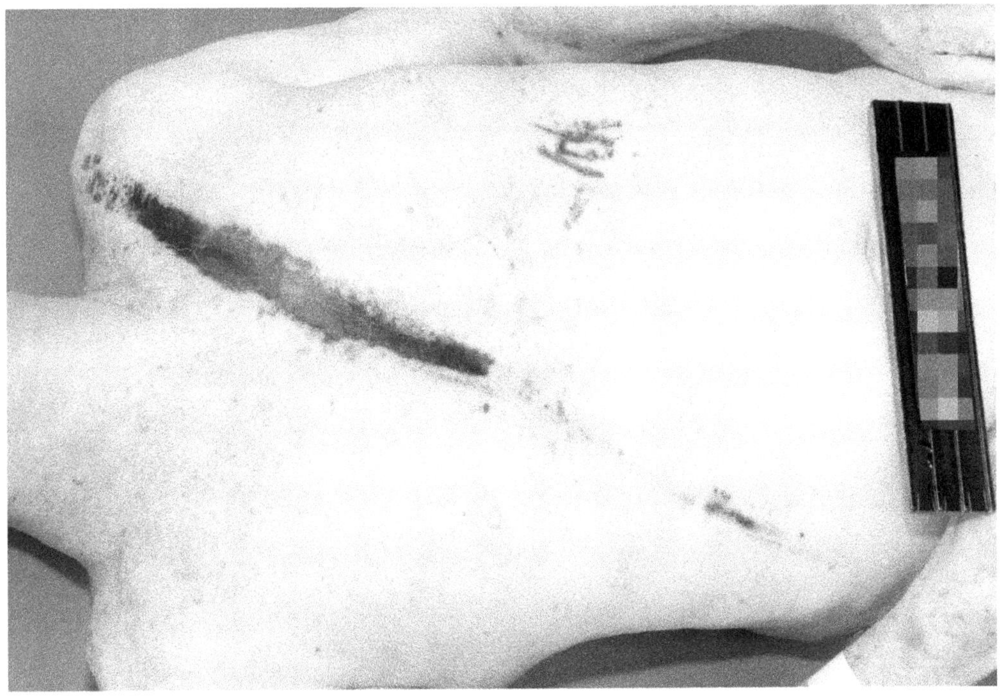

Figure 6.3 Rib spreader laceration of axilla, victim of GSW of chest with hemithoracotomy

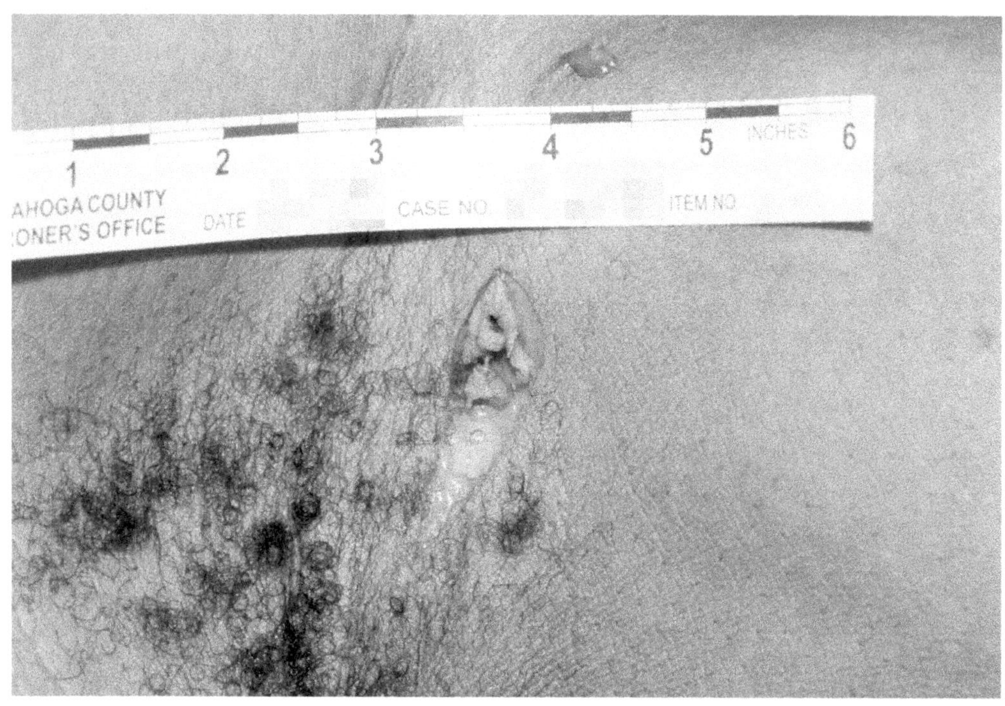

Figure 6.4 Scalp laceration with tissue bridging

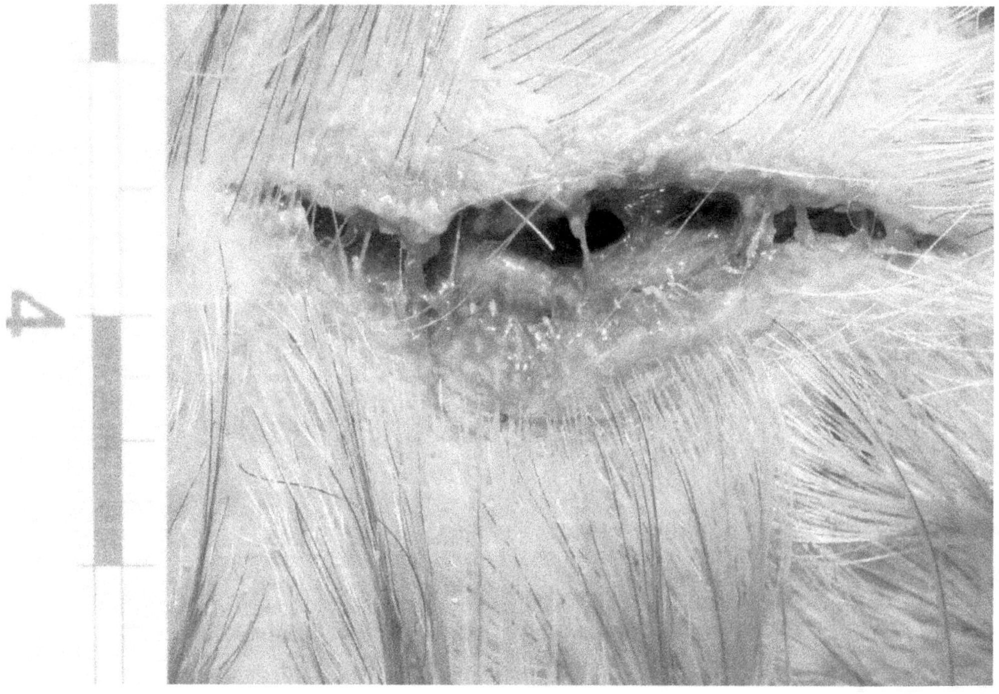

Figure 6.5 Periorbital ecchymosis arising from basal skull/supraorbital ridge fractures

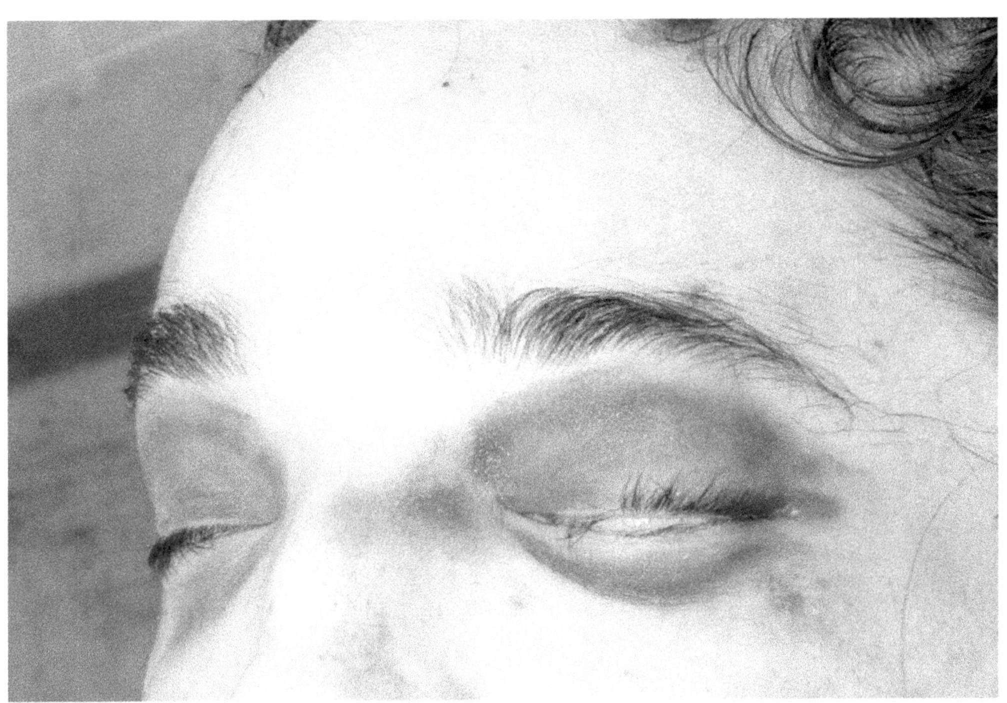

Figure 6.6 Open butterfly fracture of tibia, pedestrian victim struck by motor vehicle

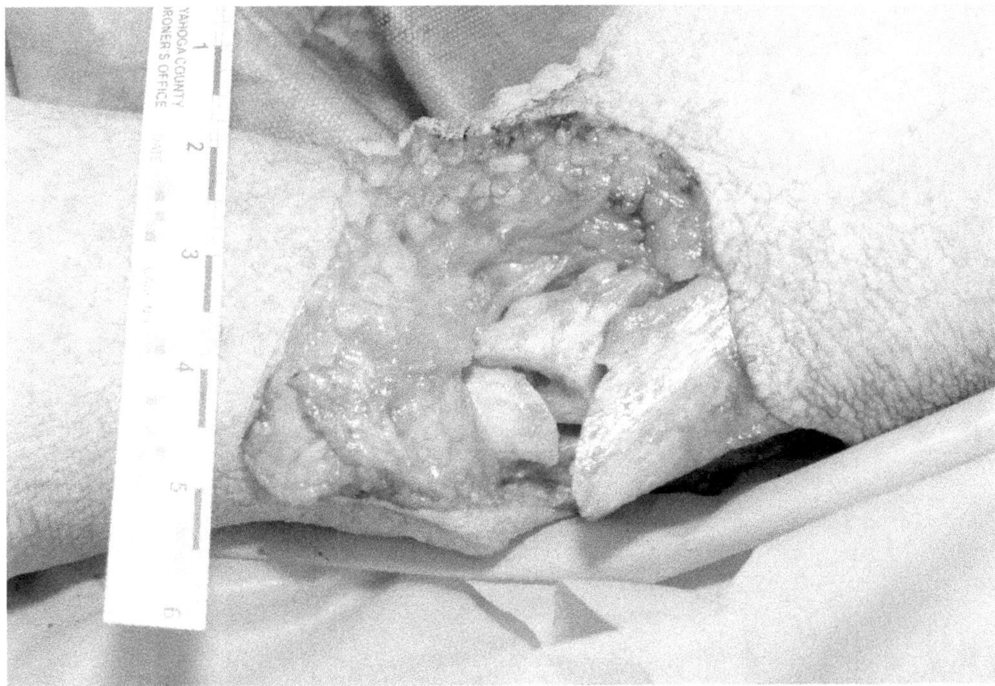

Figure 6.7 Stab wound by single-edged knife with blunting at one end (right), sutures removed

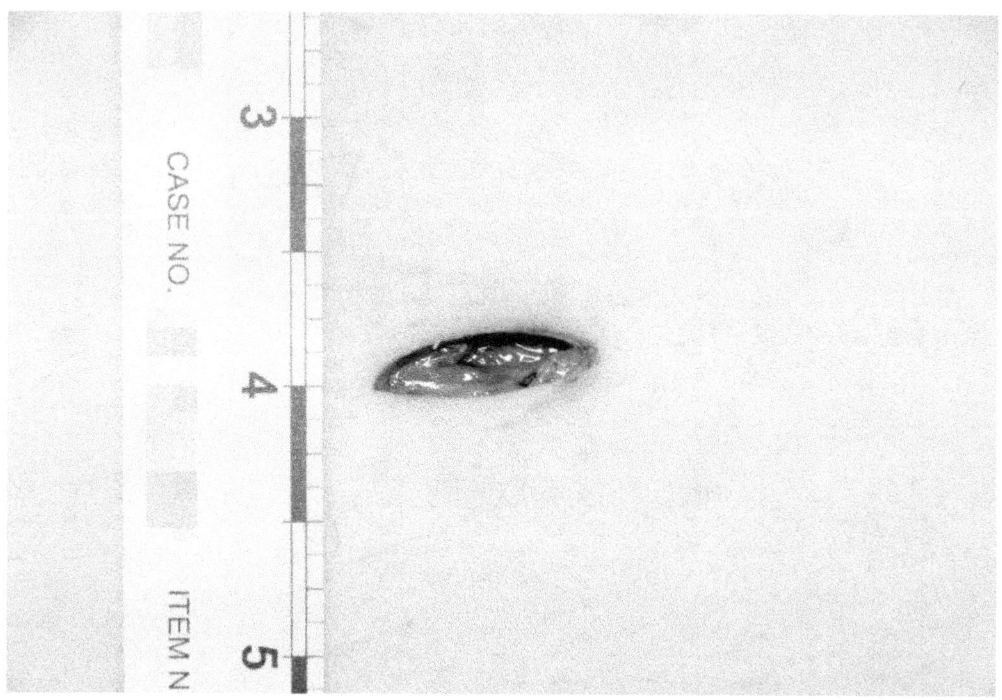

Figure 6.8 Incised wound of forearm

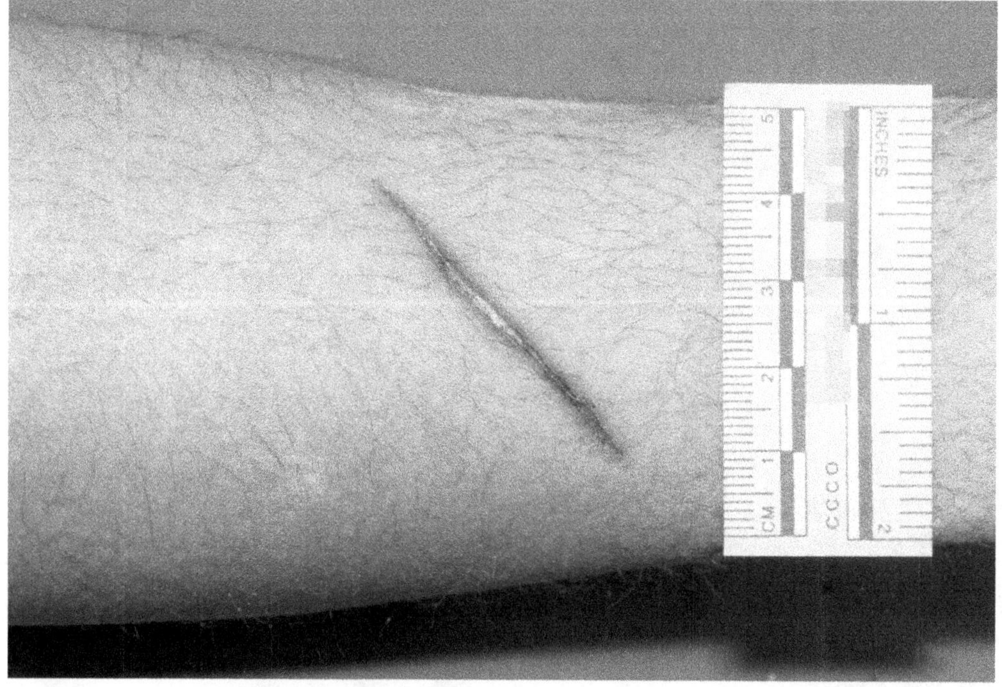

Figure 6.9 Hesitation suicidal incised wounds of forearm, healed

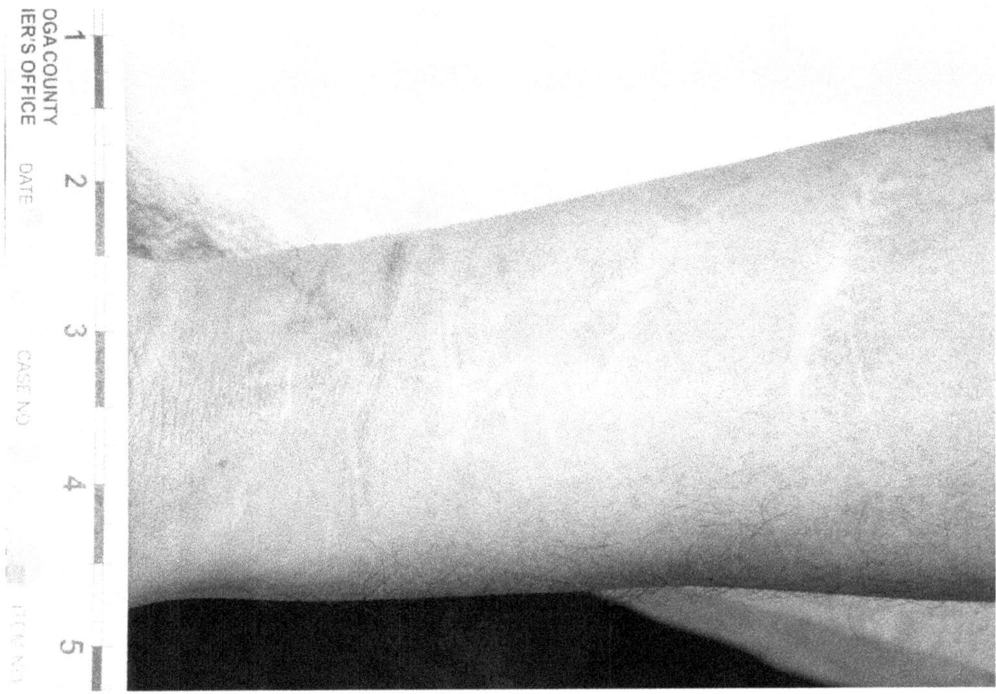

Figure 6.10 Dicing-type incised wounds from tempered glass, front seat occupant of motor vehicle collision

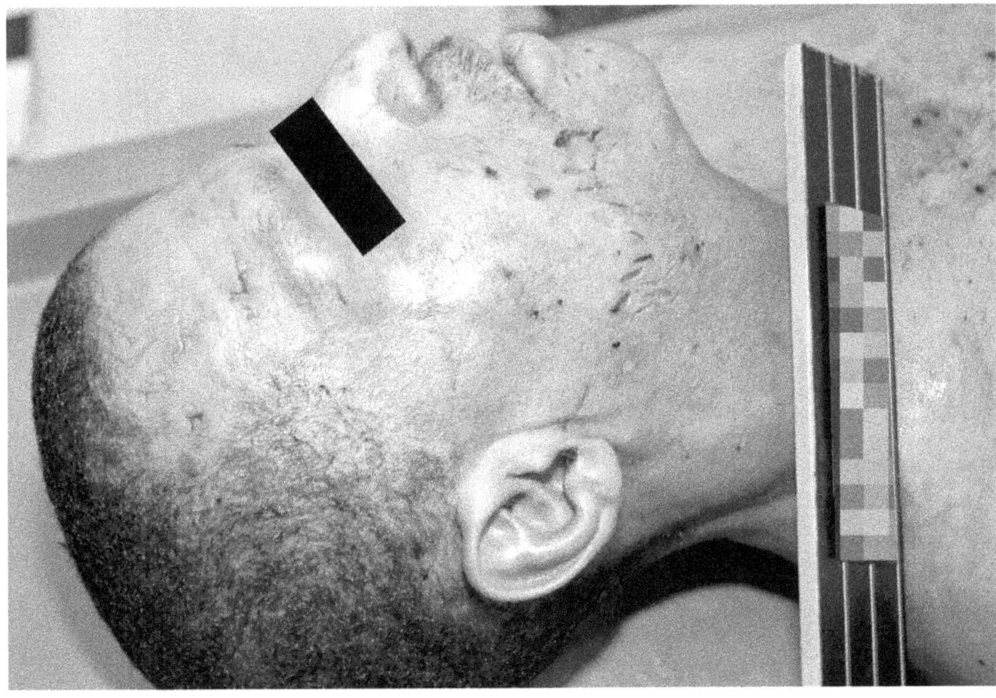

Figure 6.11 Thermal injuries from crack pipe

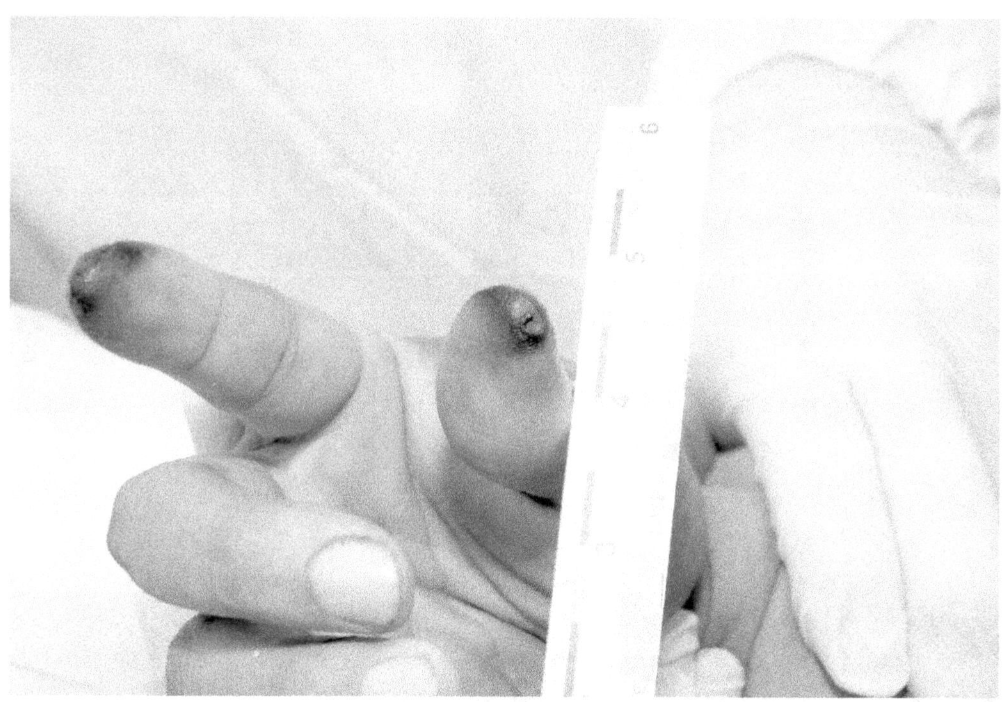

Figure 6.12 Petechial hemorrhages from resuscitative chest compressions

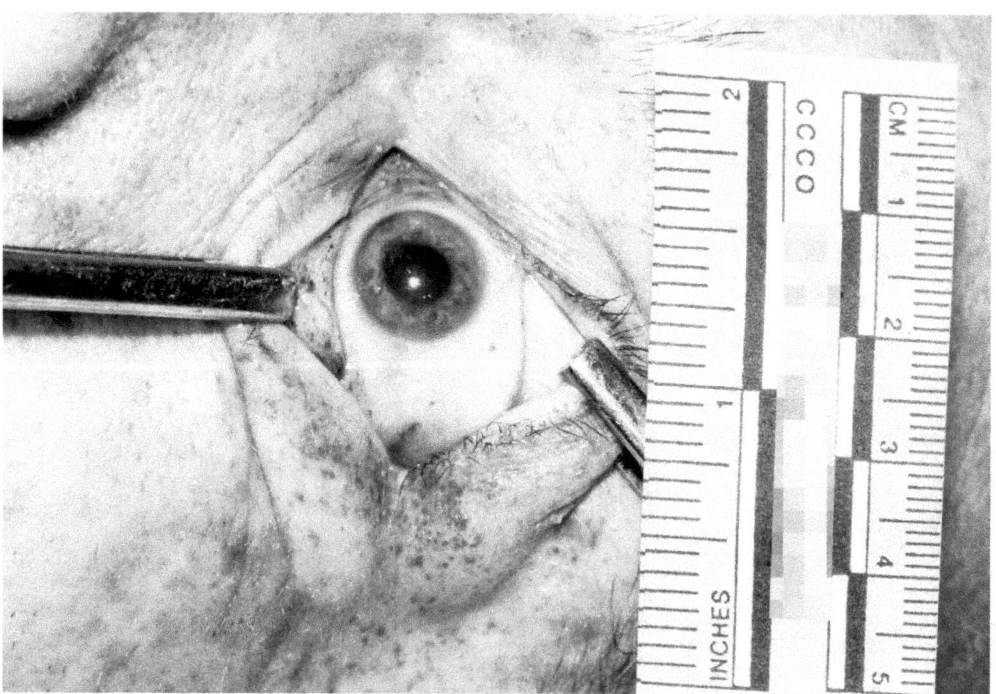

Figure 6.13 Graze type abrasion from bullet

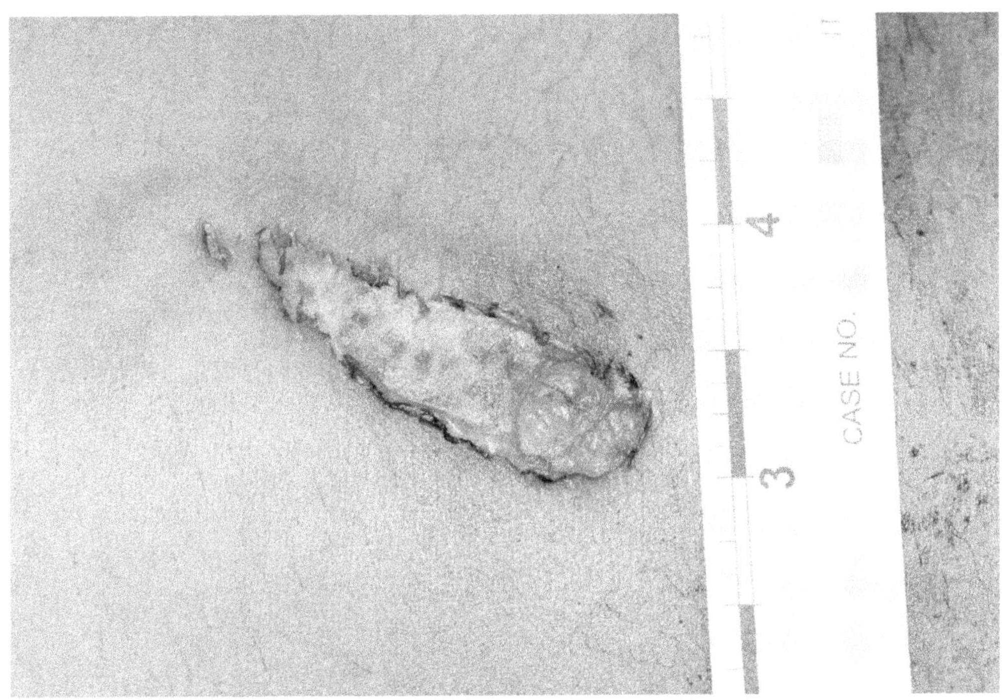

Figure 6.14 Contact entrance GSW with muzzle stamp patterned abrasion

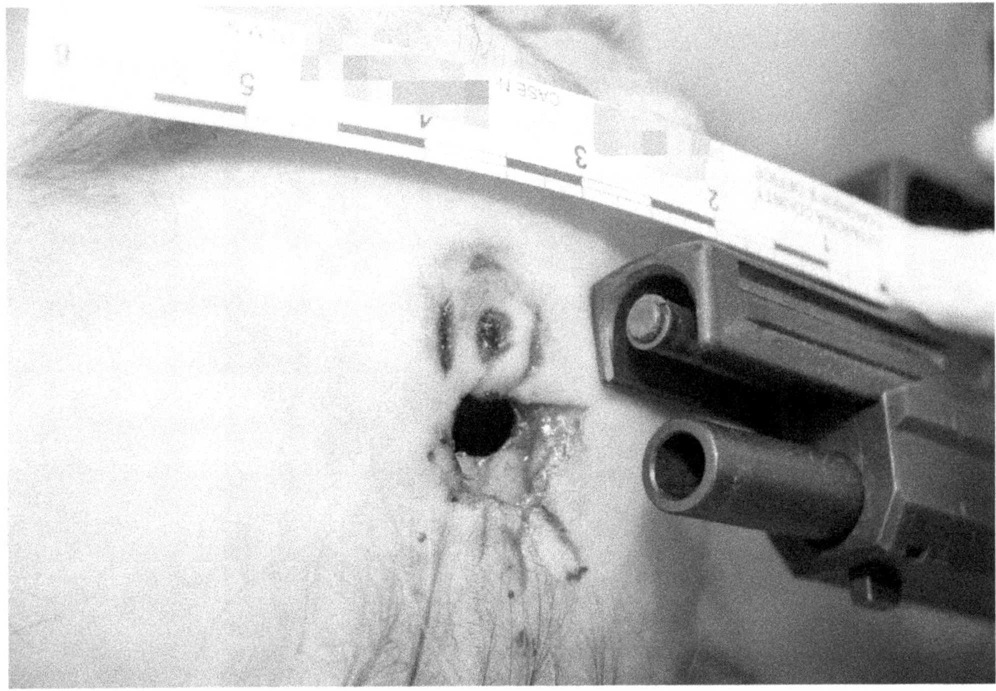

Figure 6.15 Entrance GSW with marginal and stippling abrasions

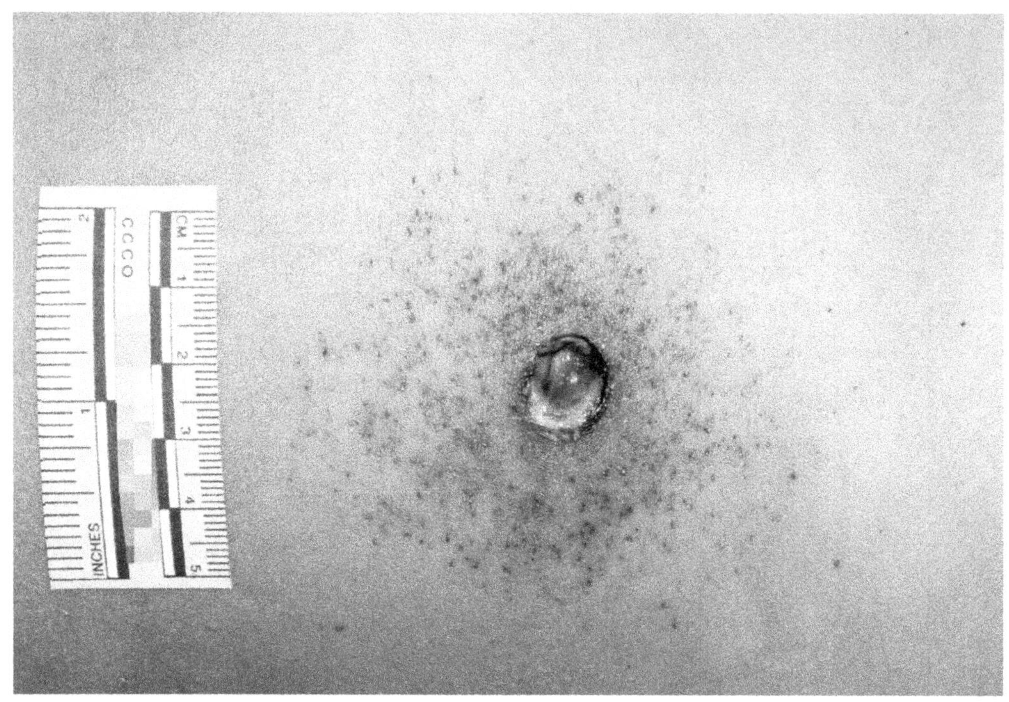

Figure 6.16 Exit GSW

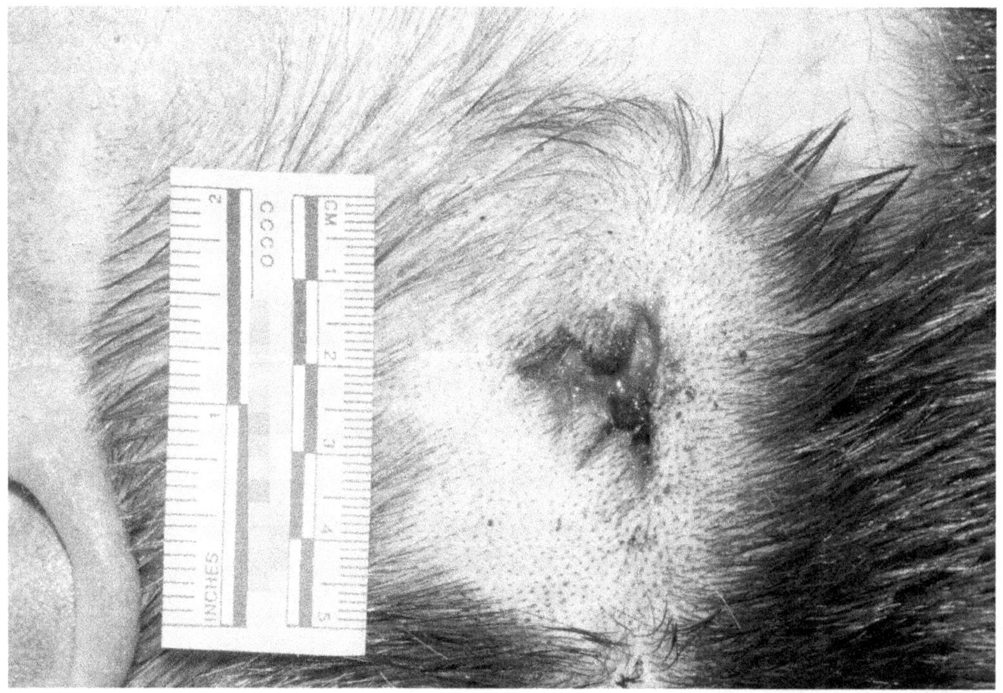

Figure 6.17 Linear track mark scar with superimposed needle punctures

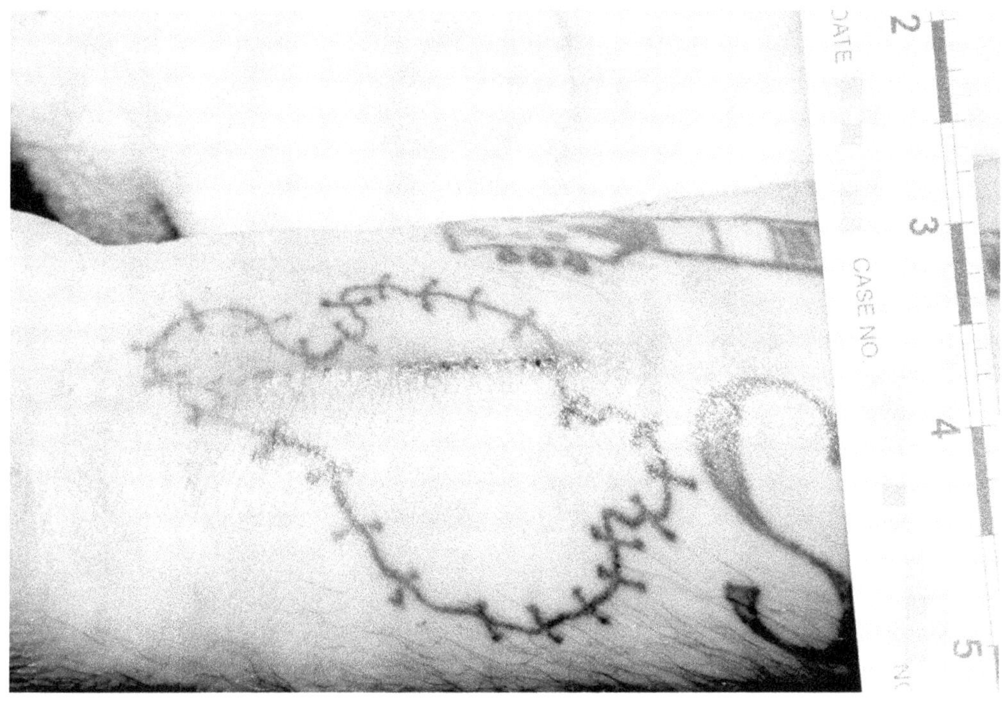

Figure 6.18 Skin popping scars

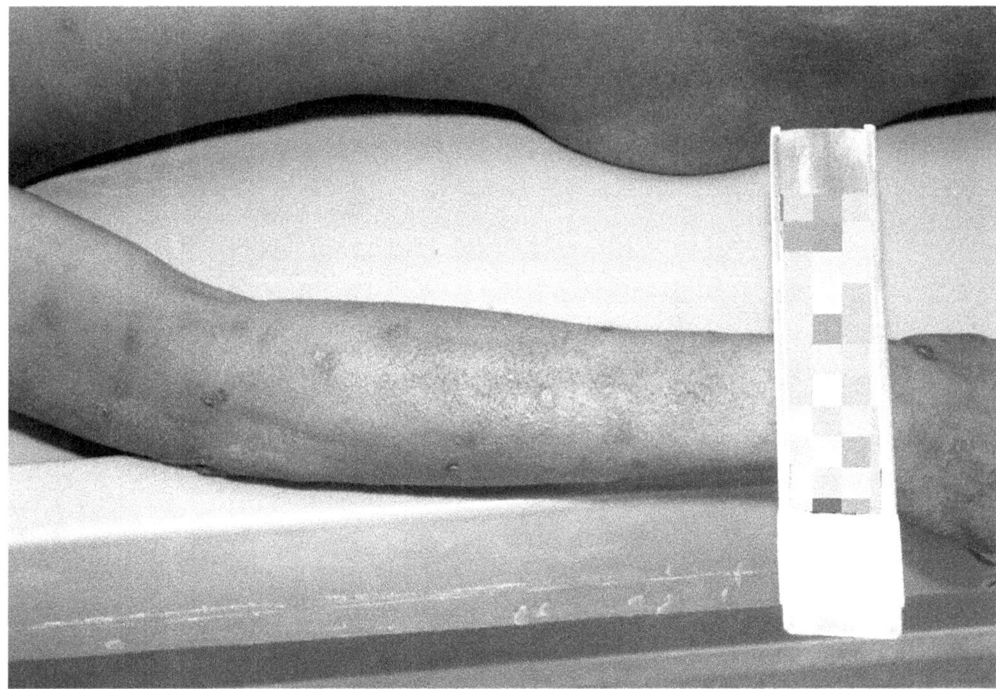

Figure 6.19 Chemical burn with drain pattern, pesticide ingestion

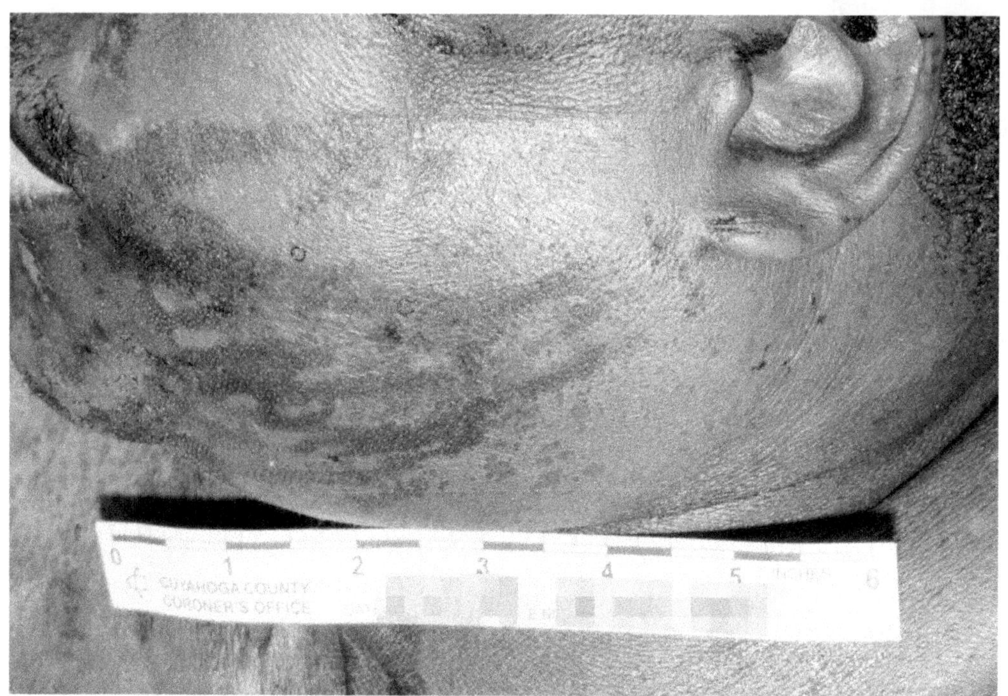

References

1. Adelson L. The forensic pathologist: "Family physician" to the bereaved. *JAMA.* 1977;237(15):1585-88.

2. Choo TM, Choi YS. Historical Development of Forensic Pathology in the United States. *Korean J Leg Med.* 2012;36:15-21.

3. Eckert W. The forensic pathology specialty certification. *Am J Forensic Med Pathol.* 1988;9(1):85-89.

4. National Institute of Standards and Technology/National Commission on Forensic Science. Increasing the number, retention, and quality of board-certified forensic pathologists. August 2015. Available at: www.justice.gov/ncfs/file/787356/download. Accessed 5/15/2016. Accessed 11/25/2016.

5. Hanzlick R. Incoming forensic pathology fellows and fellowship programs 2014-2015. Prepared for forensic pathology subcommittee of National Association of Medical Examiners. Available at: www.justice.gov/ncfs/file/787356/download. Accessed 11/25/2016.

6. Hanzlick R, Haden-Pinneri K. Forensic pathology fellowship training positions and subsequent forensic pathology work effort of past forensic pathology fellows. *Acad Forensic Pathol.* 2011;1(3):322-27.

7. Kemp WL. Forensic pathologist salaries in the United States: The results of internet data collection. *Acad Forensic Pathol.* 2014;4(4):505-13.

8. College of American Pathologists 2011 Practice Characteristics Survey. College of American Pathologists.

9. Frontline Postmortem. Death Investigation in America. Forensic Pathologists: Death Detectives. Available at: www.pbs.org/wgbh/pages/frontline/post-mortem/things-to-know/forensic-pathologists.html. Accessed 5/16/2016.

10. www.huffingtonpost.com/entry/medical-examiner-shortage-means-grieving-families-wait-months-for-results_us_5665a5fee4b079b2818f2bd6. Accessed 5/16/2016.

11. Michiue T, Ishikawa T, Quan L, et. al. Forensic pathological evaluation of injury severity and fatal outcome in traffic accidents: Five illustrative autopsy cases of clinically unexpected death. *Forensic Sci Med Pathol.* 2008;4(3):153-58.

12. http://medicalexaminer.cuyahogacounty.us/en-US/CC-HeroinInitiative.aspx. Accessed 5/29/2016.

13. Hickman MJ, Hughes KA, Strom KJ, And Ropero-Miller JD. Bureau of Justice Statistics Special Report: Medical Examiners and Coroners' Offices, 2004. Available at: www.bjs.gov/content/pub/pdf/meco04.pdf. Accessed 5/29/2016.

14. National Child Death Review Reporting System. Available at: www.childdeathreview.org. Accessed 5/20/2016.

15. Armstrong EJ. Hiding in plain sight:Clinically unrecognized fatal tooth asphyxia revealed by the forensic autopsy. *Am J Forensic Med Pathol.* 2016;31(1):14-20.

16. Collins KA and Presnell ES. Elder neglect and the pathophysiology of aging. *Am J Forensic Med Pathol.* 2007;28(2):157-62.

17. Department of Health and Human Services/National Center of Elder Abuse-Administration on Aging. Available at: www.ncea.aoa.gov/Stop_Abuse/Get_Help/State/index.aspx. Accessed 5/20/2016.

18. Bove KE, Iery C, and the Autopsy Committee College of American Pathologists. The role of the autopsy in medical malpractice cases, I-a review of 99 appeals court decisions. *Arch Pathol Lab Med.* 2002;126(9):1023-31.

19. Bove KE, Iery C, and the Autopsy Committee College of American Pathologists. The role of the autopsy in medical malpractice cases, II-controversy related to autopsy performance and reporting. *Arch Pathol Lab Med.* 2002;126(9):1032-35.

20. Pakis I, Polat O, Yayci N, and Karapirli M. Comparison of the clinical diagnosis and subsequent autopsy findings in medical malpractice. *Am J Forensic Med Pathol.* 2010;31(3):218-21.

21. Scheinfeld N, Elson DM. Delusions of parisitosis. Available at: http://emedicine.medscape.com/article/1121818-overview#a4. Accessed 6/5/2016.

Chapter 7

THE LETHAL POTENTIAL OF DISEASE

Many treated diseases, especially cardiovascular disease have the potential for sudden decompensation with sudden death. Recognition of this fact by clinicians will help allay the uncertainty and reluctance some may have in regards to certification of death. The National Center for Health Statistics' (NCHS) ranking for the leading causes of natural death lists heart disease, cancer, stroke, Alzheimer's Disease and Diabetes in the top 10 with just these few affecting multiple organ systems. Non-compliance with a prescribed medication regimen for a natural disease entity can hasten death or otherwise make it more likely. Even compliance with a prescribed medication regimen does not preclude death from certain diseases. Death due to natural disease with sudden decompensation may also occur despite therapeutic or surgical interventions such as in the case of death following exsanguination caused by an aortic aneurysmal rupture with attempted emergent reparative surgery. Sudden death by way of arrhythmia due to ischemic heart disease can occur with or without co-existent myocardial infarction or preceding signs and symptoms.

Sudden death arises out of dysfunction of one or more organs with multisystem organ effects many of which have demonstrable anatomic or clinical correlates. Others either lack entirely or have few specific anatomic and clinical findings following comprehensive analysis including review of the medical history, clinical diagnostic workup or autopsy examination. These include:

- Sudden Unexplained Infant Death (SUID)
- Sudden Infant Death Syndrome (SIDS)
- Sudden Unexpected Death in Children (SUDC)
- Sudden Adult Death Syndrome (SADS)
- Sudden Unexpected Death In Epilepsy (SUDEP)
- Sudden Unexplained Nocturnal Death Syndrome (SUNDS)

Two common threads amongst the entities listed above appear to be cardiac conduction system dysfunction with arrhythmia or central nervous system dysfunction affecting cardiac and respiratory function, with likely a genetic basis.

Diseases with lethal potential involve many organ systems and, whether predictably or unexpectedly, propagate certain physiologic derangements and non-specific processes that can terminate into cardiac arrest, respiratory arrest, or a combination of the two. Derangements, non-specific processes and conditions, terminal events, signs, and symptoms individually have limitless causes and are otherwise etiologically non-specific and as such should never appear alone as a cause of death on the death certificate (DC). Etiologic specificity is the essence of death certification as it aids in the classification of each death into a specific disease or organ system category. The etiologically specific **cause of death** is defined as the primary disease condition (or injury or intoxication) that sets off the chain of events that ultimately leads to cessation of vital function with onset of terminal events including asystole, pulseless electrical activity, and cardiac and/or respiratory arrest. These chain of events include aforementioned physiologic derangements and non-specific processes which are synonymous to the **mechanism of death.** Mechanism of death can be simply defined as *the way in which the cause of death exerts its lethal effect*. While it is unnecessary to include terminal events on the death certificate, it is permissible to include mechanisms as long as they are accompanied by the etiologically specific disease (or injury) medically known to be associated with it. Inclusion of the most prominent of the mechanisms clarifies the severity or the precipitous nature of the terminal clinical course.

The following table lists some of the more prominent non-specific disease processes/conditions, derangements, signs, and terminal events with some overlap with entities listed in Table 3.2:

Table 7.1 Selection of non-specific disease processes/conditions, derangements, signs, and terminal events (table continues onto next page)

Central/Peripheral Nervous System • Cerebral edema • Cerebral herniation • Dementia,unspecified • Encephalopathy • Hemorrhage-intracranial, intracerebral • Hydrocephalus • Intracranial hypertension • Mental status alteration, change • Neuropathy • Seizures • Status epilepticus	Cardiovascular System • Arrhythmia • Asystole • Atrial fibrillation • Bradycardia • Cardiac arrest • Cardiac tamponade • Cardiomyopathy • Coronary vasospasm • Dysrhythmia • Heart failure(acute, congestive) • Hemopericardium • Hypertension • Hypotension • Pulseless Electrical Activity (PEA) • Sudden cardiac death • Ventricular fibrillation	Respiratory System • Acute Respiratory Distress Syndrome (ARDS) • Anoxia/hypoxia • Aspiration • Atelectasis • Chronic Obstructive Pulmonary Disease (COPD) • End-stage lung disease • Hemothorax • Pleural effusion • Pneumothorax • Pulmonary edema • Pulmonary fibrosis • Pulmonary hypertension • Respiratory arrest • Respiratory failure (acute and chronic)
Gastrointestinal System • Ascites, peritoneal effusion • Cirrhosis • Diarrhea • End-stage liver disease • Hemoperitoneum • Hemorrhage -hematemesis , hematochezia • Hepatic encephalopathy • Hepatic failure • Hepatorenal syndrome • Intestinal obstruction • Peritonitis • Portal hypertension	Hematologic/immune/ infectious • Anemia • Bacteremia • Coagulopathy • Cytopenias • Disseminated Intravascular Coagulation (DIC) • Hemolysis • Hemorrhage • Leukocytosis • Sepsis/Septic shock • Systemic Inflammatory Response Syndrome (SIRS)	Renal System • Chronic kidney disease • Oliguria • Polyuria • Renal failure (acute and chronic) • Uremia

Endocrine System	Musculoskeletal	Multisystem, System non-specific
• Adrenal crisis • Diabetes insipidus • Thyrotoxicosis • Hypopituitarism	• Cellulitis • Decubital/pressure ulcers • Fasciitis • Gangrene	• Acid/base disorders (acidosis, alkalosis) • Anaphylaxis/ anaphylactoid reaction • Carcinomatosis • Dehydration • Electrolyte disturbance (hyper/hyponatremia, hyper/hypokalemia,hyper/hypo glycemia) • Hyperpyrexia • Hyperthermia • Hypothermia • Hypovolemia • Malnutrition • Multiple system organ failure/dysfunction • Neoplasia • Paraneoplastic syndromes • Shock

Disease mechanisms and non-specific disease conditions are rooted in physiologic dysfunction and loss of regulatory mechanisms, from the subcellular molecular level to the organ system level. When each mechanism or condition is examined individually, a differential list of causal entities can be enumerated. For example, hypoxia may be the effect of respiratory failure due to pulmonary arterial thromboembolism arising from deep vein thrombosis, heroin overdose, or fat embolism associated with long bone fracture. The clinical workup of a patient with hypoxia would address a list of differential diagnoses generated in the context of the clinical history and presentation, in search of the specific underlying cause(s) as the treatments for each could be very different. A similar approach applies for the purpose of death certification of a death involving terminal hypoxia whereby listing hypoxia alone on the death certificate would be insufficient as a cause of death as it provides no information as to what led to it. Hypoxia is also associated with number of other disease conditions, trauma, and medical procedures. For the purposes of generating mortality data derived from cause-of-death information, a death involving terminal hypoxia caused by one type of disease (or injury) would be classified differently than hypoxia caused by a different type of disease (or injury).

Many disease conditions with lethal potential are diagnosable clinically and many of them manifest with structural alterations making them identifiable grossly, microscopically, and increasingly on a molecular level. Some diseases like epilepsy or cardiac disease caused by channelopathies often have little or no demonstrable structural pathology and therefore the medical record or other historical information becomes the focus in the search for an etiology. The clinical and pathological approach to identifying the etiologically specific medical cause leading to a particular death facilitates more precise death certification. It is recognized that at times while the pathophysiologic changes may be clinically known, the etiologic agent or condition remains unknown, uncertain, or has not been completely elucidated at the time of death. It is permissible to indicate uncertainty or probability on the death certificate in those instances.

Table 7.2 lists a selection of major disease conditions with lethal potential and corresponding select mechanisms and processes of death.

Table 7.2 Select system-specific disease conditions with lethal potential and some corresponding mechanisms (*indicates conditions also associated with other *underlying* disease conditions, trauma, intoxicants, or environmental causes)

Central and Peripheral Nervous Systems:

Arterial aneurysmal rupture	Mass effect, vasospasm, hemorrhage, ischemia, infarction, hydrocephalus
Arterial atherosclerotic stenosis or thrombosis with infarct	Cerebral edema, herniation, cardiopulmonary arrest
Bacterial meningitis	Vasculitis, ischemia, cerebral edema, hydrocephalus
* Dementias-neurodegenerative and vascular types	Cerebral atrophy, encephalopathy, various sequela associated with loss of cognition and mobility, failure to thrive
*Encephalopathy and encephalitis	Edema, seizures, hydrocephalus
*Guillian-Barre Syndrome	Pneumonia, respiratory failure, sepsis, venous thrombosis, autonomic instability
*Hypertensive hemorrhage (stroke)	Cerebral edema, herniation, intraventricular hemorrhage, hydrocephalus, ischemia, infarction
Malignant neoplasms	Seizures, cerebral edema, ventricular obstruction, herniation, paraneoplastic syndr.
Multiple Sclerosis	Sequela of autonomic, sympathetic and parasympathetic dysfunction
*Seizure disorder/epilepsy	Encephalopathy, arrhythmia, hypoxia, cardiorespiratory failure

(Table 7.2 continued)

Cardiovascular System:

Alcoholic cardiomyopathy	Arrhythmia, heart failure
Anomalous origin of coronary artery	Myocardial ischemia, arrhythmia
Atherosclerotic cardiovascular/coronary artery disease	Plaque rupture with thrombosis/occlusion and myocardial infarction, vasospasm, ischemic myocardial fibrosis, arrhythmia
Bacterial, fungal endocarditis	Valvular stenosis, insufficiency, embolization
*Cardiomyopathy (ex. hypertrophic, dilated, ischemic, amyloidosis, sarcoidosis, radiation-induced, hemochromatosis)	Myocardial ischemic fibrosis, arrhythmia, heart failure
Cardiomyopathy, other (restrictive, arrhythmogenic right/left ventricular dysplasia, left ventricular non-compaction)	Arrhythmia, heart failure
Channelopathies (ex. Long QT syndrome, catecholaminergic polymorphic ventricular tachycardia CPVT)	Arrhythmia, heart failure
*Coronary arterial dissection	Myocardial ischemia, infarction, vasospasm, arrhythmia
*Drug-associated cardiac toxicity (ex. cocaine, ethanol, anthracycline)	Myocardial hypertrophy, ischemic fibrosis, heart failure, arrhythmia
Hypertensive cardiovascular disease	Myocardial hypertrophy, ischemic fibrosis, arrhythmia, heart failure
Myocarditis (viral, bacterial)	Arrhythmia, heart failure
*Myocardial infarction, acute	Wall rupture with hemopericardium and tamponade, papillary muscle rupture with insufficiency, heart failure, arrhythmia
Valvular heart disease-annular calcification	Arrhythmia, heart failure
Valvular heart disease-congenitally bicuspid aortic valve	Stenosis, heart failure, aortic dissection
Valvular heart disease-mitral valve prolapse, aortic stenosis	Ventricular hypertrophy, ischemic fibrosis, arrhythmia, heart failure

(Table 7.2 continued)

Vascular-non cardiac:

Arterial fibromuscular dysplasia	Organ ischemia, infarction, or dysfunction
*Aortic dissection with/without rupture (Types A and B)	Stroke, myocardial infarction, GI infarct, renal infarction, exsanguination
*Aortic aneurysmal rupture	Exsanguination
*Cerebral artery aneurysm rupture (spontaneous)	Ischemic/hemorrhagic infarction, hydrocephalus
*Mesenteric artery thrombosis	Bowel ischemia, infarction, perforation, peritonitis, infection
Vascular malformations and proliferations- arteriovenous, hemangiomas, varices	Hemorrhage
Vasculitides	Various sequela of end-organ dysfunction including ischemic infarct, hemorrhage, and thrombosis

Respiratory System:

*COPD- Asthma	Airway obstruction with asphyxia, hypoxia, respiratory failure
COPD- Obesity/obstructive sleep apnea hypoventilation syndrome	Hypoxia, pulmonary hypertension, pulmonary hemorrhage, pulmonary fibrosis, respiratory and heart failure
*COPD- Pulmonary emphysema	Hypoxia, respiratory failure, pulmonary hypertension, pneumothorax, heart failure
*Epiglottitis, laryngitis, tracheitis	Airway edema and obstruction with asphyxia
*Pneumonia (bacterial, viral, bronchial, lobar)	Pulmonary hemorrhage, edema, effusion, hypoxia, asphyxia, respiratory failure
*Pulmonary embolism (thrombus, fat ,bone marrow, air)	Heart failure, ventilation/perfusion mismatch, hypoxia
Malignant neoplasia	Hemorrhage, post-obstructive pneumonia, hypoxia, respiratory failure, paraneoplastic sequela
Sarcoidosis	Fibrosis, hypoxia, respiratory failure, hemorrhage
Tuberculosis	Hemorrhage

(Table 7.2 continued)

Gastrointestinal System:

*Acute pancreatitis	Systemic inflammatory reaction, cardiovascular, respiratory, and renal failure
Alcoholic liver disease	Metabolic and electrolyte derangements, encephalopathy
*Bacterial colitis	Diarrhea with electrolyte, fluid, and acid/base disturbances
*Gastric ulcer erosion/perforation	Hemorrhage
*Hepatic cirrhosis	Liver failure, portal hypertension, GI hemorrhage, coagulopathy, encephalopathy
*Intestinal infarction	Rupture with peritonitis, sepsis
*Intestinal obstruction, incarceration, strangulation	Ischemia, infarction, rupture with peritonitis, sepsis
Malignant neoplasm	Obstruction, hemorrhage, paraneoplastic sequela
Non-alcoholic steatosis/steatohepatitis	Metabolic derangement
Peptic ulcer erosion/perforation	Hemorrhage
*Ruptured varix	Hemorrhage

Genitourinary System:

Acute pyelonephritis	Bacteremia, sepsis, septic shock
Intrinsic renal diseases (nephritides, nephrosis)	Sequela of fluid and electrolyte disturbance, red cell production, protein metabolism, excretion of waste products, renal failure, hypertension and sequela
Malignancy: renal, bladder, prostate, testicular, uterine, endometrial, ovarian, cervical	Various sequela including metastasis and paraneoplastic syndromes, surgical complications, chemotherapeutic complications
Ruptured ectopic pregnancy	Hemorrhage
Ruptured corpus luteum cyst	Hemorrhage
*Urinary tract infection with urosepsis	Various sequela of sepsis

(Table 7.2 continued)

Endocrine System:

Autoimmune polyglandular syndromes	Various sequela of glandular hypofunction (ex. adrenal insufficiency)
Grave's Disease	Sequela of thyrotoxicosis
Insulin Dependent Diabetes Mellitus (primary or secondary)	Ketoacidosis, dehydration, hyperkalemia, cerebral edema, Acute Respiratory Distress Syndrome
Non-insulin Dependent Diabetes Mellitus	Non-ketotic hyperosmolar sequela

Hemolymphatic System and Infectious:

Acute leukemia, lymphoma	Coagulopathy, organ dysfunction and rupture, paraneoplastic syndromes, infectious disease complications
Human Immunodeficiency Virus/Acquired Immunodeficiency Syndrome	Sequela of opportunistic infections and malignancies
*Organism specific bacterial, fungal, and viral infections	Sepsis, septic embolization, systemic inflammatory reaction, secondary infection, sequela of chronic infection or post-inflammatory changes
Viral influenza	Respiratory failure, secondary bacterial pneumonia
Sickle Cell Disease	Thromboembolism, hemolysis, sequela of end-organ damage, bacterial sepsis, marrow failure, hemolysis

Pregnancy-associated:

Cardiomyopathy	Cardiac failure
*Placental abruption and accreta	Coagulopathy, hemorrhage
Pre-eclampsia/Eclampsia	Encephalopathy, cerebral hemorrhage, seizures, cardiac failure, hepatic failure, hepatic rupture, coagulopathy with hemorrhage
Ruptured cerebral artery aneurysm	Mass effect, vasospasm, ischemia, infarction, hydrocephalus
Sheehan's Syndrome, lymphocytic hypophysitis	Variable sequela of pituitary gland hypofunction

(Table 7.2 continued)

Fetal/Infant:

Congenital adrenal hyperplasia-associated enzyme deficiencies	Electrolyte deficiencies, hypotension, dehydration, hypoglycemia
Congenital bacterial and viral pneumonia	Hypoxia, sepsis, multi-organ system effects
Congenital heart diseases (Tetralogy of Fallot, atrial and ventricular septal defect, pulmonary atresia, aortic coarctation, anomalous pulmonary venous return)	Hypoxia, cardiac and respiratory failure
*Germinal matrix hemorrhage	Seizures, multi-organ system effects, developmental delay
*Hemolytic disease of the newborn	Kernicterus, hydrops, neurological sequela
Inborn errors of metabolism	Various systemic effects
Infectious (TORCH infections, parvovirus B19, varicella zoster virus, listeria)	Multi-organ system effects
*Necrotizing enterocolitis	Perforation, peritonitis, sepsis
*Respiratory distress syndrome/hyaline membrane disease	Hypoxia, respiratory failure

Miscellaneous:

*Anaphylaxis /anaphylactoid reaction	Cardiovascular, respiratory failure
Chronic alcoholism/ethanolism	Multi-organ system pathology: brain, heart, lungs, liver, blood vessels, GI tract, peripheral nervous system, nutritional, metabolic, electrolyte
Chronic drug/medication insufflation	Chronic lung disease with respiratory failure, cardiomyopathy with heart failure
Chronic intravenous drug/medication abuse	Endocarditis, bacterial sepsis, chronic lung disease with respiratory failure, cardiomyopathy with heart failure
Malignant neoplasms (breast, lung, GI, neuroendocrine, hemolymphatic)	Paraneoplastic syndromes including hypercoagulation with thromboembolism, sequela of radiation, chemotherapy, and surgery
Multivisceral sarcoidosis	Multiple organ effects, especially lungs and heart
*Neuroleptic malignant syndrome; serotonin syndrome	Effects of institution, withdrawal or co-administration of drugs and medications

Aside from neuroleptic malignant syndrome listed above, a number of other syndromes are medically known to have lethal potential usually encompassing a constellation of disease conditions with varied and overlapping symptomatology, that give rise to other variable intervening disease conditions and complications as a result of physiologic derangement(s) caused. For others, the specific underlying cause is unknown. For some of these syndromes, the underlying cause may involve toxins, medications, or injury. Therefore, deaths arising from certain syndromes must be reported to the medical examiner or coroner. Examples of syndromes with lethal potential include the following (* indicates possible underlying non-natural cause):

- Acquired Immunodeficiency Syndrome (AIDS)
- *Acute compartment syndrome
- Brugada Syndrome
- *Central Cord Syndrome (CCS)
- *Drug-induced serotonin syndrome
- Ehlers-Danlos Syndrome
- *Hepatorenal Syndrome
- Marfan Syndrome
- Mitochondrial Myopathy Encephalopathy Lactic Acidosis Stroke (MELAS)
- Polyglandular autoimmune syndrome Type II
- Paraneoplastic syndromes

Many of the disease conditions appearing in table 7.2 arise from a number of specific underlying, medically linked, causative or associated disease conditions, trauma, intoxication, or envenomation. For example, encephalopathy may be caused by malignant hypertension, complications of acute and chronic ethanol intoxication, infections, toxins, insect venom, or the sequela of head trauma. Intractable diarrhea associated with bacterial colitis caused by *Clostridium* bacteria may follow antibiotic treatment for iatrogenic or trauma-associated infection. Anaphylaxis may be the result of exposure to a specific food allergen, insect venom, or intravenous contrast media. The aim during the normal course of clinical evaluation of the patient is to elucidate the underlying cause (s) most importantly for treatment purposes and also for updating the list of medical conditions in the medical record later to be coded using the ICD-CM coding system.

In the determination of the cause of death by way of autopsy, the pathologist must evaluate all disease (and injury) findings in the context of any medical history and/or clinical findings and select the condition most incompatible with life. In forensic pathology practice, a 5-tier classification scheme is utilized to facilitate determination of the cause of death. This classification scheme ranks the lethal potential of disease demonstrable at autopsy and/or on clinical grounds and is summarized below along with illustrative examples [1]:

- **Class I**: demonstrable pathology or lethal mechanism incompatible with vital function to a degree of absolute certainty; ex. spontaneous acute rupture of ascending aortic dissection with hemopericardium and cardiac tamponade

- **Class II:** demonstrable advanced pathology with lethal potential but without the additional presence of catastrophic complication(s) that would qualify as Class I; ex. moderate to severe atherosclerotic coronary artery stenosis, cardiomegaly, focal acute myocardial ischemic changes, and patchy myocardial fibrosis in decedent with a history of unstable angina

- **Class III**: demonstrable marginal pathology deemed insufficient to cause death but with compelling history and no other competing causes; ex. moderate atherosclerotic coronary artery stenosis with acute intraplaque hemorrhage and a history of sudden death shortly following exertional activity

- **Class IV**: functional, non-structural pathology that would otherwise be clinically evident, with compelling history of symptoms, and with absence of competing causes; ex. Non-traumatic Seizure Disorder/epilepsy with history of increased seizure frequency, medication non-compliance, and subtherapeutic anti-seizure medication blood levels found on postmortem analysis

- **Class V**: competent autopsy performance with microscopic, toxicology, and chemistry analyses and evaluation of all available history fail to elucidate a cause of death; the cause of death in this instance would be listed as "undetermined"

The principles of this classification scheme are also applicable to natural deaths occurring in medical facilities and may be useful to hospital pathologists and clinicians involved in the synthesis of autopsy information and in the certification of these types of deaths.

References

1. Adams VI, Flomenbaum MA, and Hirsch CS. 2006. Trauma and Disease. In *Medicolegal investigation of death-Guidelines for the application of pathology to crime scene investigation.* Ed. WU Spitz, 447-49. 4th ed. Springfield, IL: Charles C Thomas Publisher Ltd.

Chapter 8

THE CLINICIAN CERTIFIER OF DEATH

Introduction

Certification of death is the act of entering the medical cause of death by the certifier in the appropriate section of the death certificate. The **certifier of death** is the clinical physician, physician medical examiner, or the coroner. In some locales, the nurse practitioner, physician assistant, dentist, or chiropractor is authorized to be the certifier. **The Centers for Disease Control and Prevention's (CDC) Model State Vital Statistics Act expressly defines the certifying primary or attending physician as the physician who treated the decedent within the 12 months preceding the death or his/her associate physician, the chief medical officer of the institution, or the physician who performed the autopsy** [1] (i.e. the hospital pathologist). The statutes of each state redefine and clarify who can be the certifier of death. Fully licensed physicians (as opposed to those with trainee certificates) are included in this category. Not in every locale is a medically trained individual required to certify the death. For example, in some rural jurisdictions within the state of Texas, the Justice of the Peace or a judge by law can certify the death. While medical examiners and coroners certify deaths on a very regular basis, they only certify approximately 20% of the Nation's deaths, aligned with the percentage of jurisdictional deaths investigated. This includes clinician-certified death certificates amended by the ME/C because of wording in the cause-of-death statement indicative of non-natural conditions or complications of injury. Thus, **the majority of deaths, approximately 80%, are certified by those in clinical practice**. For clinical practitioners, end-of-life care does not simply end with pronouncement of death and notification of the family. Death certification too is a patient care duty and a final courtesy to your patient.

Clinicians certify only natural deaths. Deaths associated with significant injury, poisoning or intoxication or that are work-related must be reported to the ME/C, who will certify those deaths. Deaths arising from known or suspected complications of therapy or surgery are reportable and the clinician would not certify these deaths once/if jurisdiction is assumed by the ME/C. Deaths associated with insignificant injury acquired accidentally, in the context of significant natural disease with lethal potential *are* certifiable by clinicians. By application of the "but for" principle, that but for the presence of minor accidental injury, in the setting of natural disease with lethal potential, the patient would have died at approximately the same time. Deaths in which there is a recent history of injury due to an assault, especially if the injured person was not medically evaluated and had an interval of survival, should not be certified by clinicians and instead must be reported to the ME/C.

The **death certificate (DC)** is a legal document and proof of death. It is a formalized tracking system for the many different causes of death and associated demographics. It is one of several vital records (the others being birth, marriage, divorce, and fetal death certificates) used not only to document a significant and final earthly human milestone but also for the derivation of statistical data. A multitude of federal, state, and other local agencies utilize statistical data derived from death certificates to facilitate epidemiological study, health monitoring, healthcare fund allocation, law-making, and social and medical research. **Therefore, the optimization of the Nation's overall health is largely dependent upon the quality of information entered on DCs.** As part of the national vital data program called the National Vital Statistics System (NVSS) with the guidelines put forth by the CDC's National Center for Health Statistics (NCHS), the **U.S. Standard Certificate of Death** shown in Figure 8.1 is the basic format used by the States to collect demographic and cause-of-death information on their own modified versions. The disease and/or injury as listed under the cause-of-death section on the death certificate is read, analyzed, and coded using the International Statistical Classification of Diseases and Health Related Problems system currently in its 10th edition (ICD-10).

There are misconceptions regarding death certification that need addressing as they ultimately lead to the delay in certification, which is distinctly a disservice to the decedent's family or the decedent's legal guardian and to public health surveillance efforts. These include:

- Completion/signing of the DC is unimportant
- The local Medical Examiner/Coroner is responsible for completing and signing all DCs clinicians fail to complete
- Only the attending physician can complete and sign a DC
- There are no consequences for a clinician who fails to complete/sign a DC
- The clinician will be penalized if the listed cause of death is incorrect

First, the consequences resulting from uncompleted death certificates have widespread ramifications ranging from delayed funeral proceedings to adverse financial and emotional hardship on the bereaved family to lags in updated public health information. To the second and third points, it is the responsibility of the treating physician or authorized designated clinical practitioner who has knowledge regarding a patient's health condition(s) and/or the terminal clinical course to certify any death that does not fall under the jurisdiction of the ME/C. This would also include the physician in attendance at the time of the death (the pronouncing physician) but does not preclude other treating physicians, senior residents, or authorized clinical practitioners as defined in the Introduction. Fourthly, state law requires that DCs be registered within a mandated time period of up to 5 days from the date of death and clinicians are required to certify the death within 2 to 3 days of receipt of notification from funeral director. Failure to certify a death is not completely without consequence and disciplinary action inclusive of fines, license suspension, and license revocation can be enacted by state medical boards in accordance with statutes. Concerned parties including families and funeral directors who do not receive a DC or encounter delay of the same may be inclined to report the responsible clinician to the state medical board resulting in investigation and disciplinary action. Finally, while the death certificate itself is a legal document that verifies the event of death, the medical cause of death listed on this document is an *opinion* based on known medical information at the time of the death and is *not* a guarantee of accuracy. It is the certifier's best educated guess that in all probability (more likely than not or greater than 50% certainty) that the patient expired as a result of the listed cause of death. This level of certainty is much less than the degree of medical certainty that has been required when stating an expert medical opinion in court, during a deposition, or on a written report. Furthermore, there is no penalty for an incorrect cause-of-death opinion that was made in good faith on the basis of known information at the time of the death. Should that opinion change as a result of unexpected findings arising from pre-mortem clinical testing received *after* certification of the death or upon receipt and review of autopsy-related testing, the death certificate can be amended.

The certification of death should not conjure up thoughts of disdain or aversion. The astute clinician possesses the knowledge and wherewithal to render the best informed medical opinion that succinctly provides the reason for the patient's demise. The clinician has first-hand knowledge of the patient's disease condition(s) and can more quickly access clinical records and diagnostic test results than can the local ME/C. Unfortunately, despite the importance of death certification, clinician trainees receive very little instruction and in-service didactic lectures may be far and few between or non-existent altogether. Hence, a major goal of this publication is to bridge the knowledge gap as it pertains to proper death certification.

The addition of regularly scheduled didactic lectures and online exercises that can be counted as educational credit, inclusion of death certification questions on resident in-service examinations, and the inclusion of death certification proficiency as a core competency/milestone requirement are additional ways that teaching medical facilities can ensure that physicians gain competency and remain competent in death certification. Questions regarding death reporting and death certification should also be included on the clinical specialty board examinations. Regularly scheduled morbidity and mortality conferences should also include follow-up and review of the death certificates generated on deaths occurring on arrival, after arrival, and during hospitalization, especially those deaths that have fallen under the jurisdiction of the ME/C. Conference participants could include ME/C pathologists who certified deaths originating from the hospital. Alternatively, a resident could be delegated to contact the ME/C's office to obtain cause-of-death information on relevant cases which would add a unique educational dimension. Optimally, a memorandum of understanding between residency training programs in the primary care specialties and the local medical examiner or coroner's office should be established along with academic appointment and provision of stipends for the forensic pathology staff who would serve as key participants in the educational process pertaining to death reporting and death certification.

Before commencing to certify a death, it is necessary to familiarize oneself with the death certificate and make certain preparations prior to completing it.

8.1 The Death Certificate: Origins and Composition

The origin of death registration and statistical derivation of death information dates back many centuries starting in mid-15th century Italy and spreading to other European countries with the development boards of health [2].

The need to monitor disease epidemics and develop preventative strategies through scientific advancement spurred this evolution.

Death registration in the United States, like death investigation, has its origins in England with the first death registration law enacted by Massachusetts in 1842. The American Medical Association (AMA) was instrumental in prompting legislative bodies to establish offices for the registration of vital events inclusive of deaths. By 1900, 10 states and the District of Columbia were collecting mortality statistics extending to all states by 1933. Death registration is done at the state level following the standards and guidelines set by the Division of Vital Statistics within the CDC's National Center for Health Statistics (NCHS). The NCHS publishes the **U.S. Standard Certificate of Death** (US DC) as a standard format for the collection of death data and associated demographic data which since the early 1900s has undergone multiple revisions, approximately every 10 years. The inclusion of a pregnancy status item, more detailed how-to instructions, a tobacco use item, and minor modifications of other items appear in the most recent 2003 version. Medical associations with a vested interest in and whom have made significant contributions and recommendations for the versions of the US DC include the American Medical Association (AMA), the National Association of Medical Examiners (NAME), the College of American Pathologists (CAP} and the American Hospital Association (AHA). The US DC is based on the international medical certificate of causes of death put forth by the World Health Organization (WHO), an agency of the United Nations (UN), thereby facilitating international health comparisons. Each individual state agrees to use the US DC as the model upon which to base their DCs for the uniform collection of death information from which the NCHS can extract and compile statistical data for the purpose of not only interstate health comparisons but also for international health comparisons inclusive of the signatories of WHO. While there are slight variations relative to the content and length of the DCs between states, the overall composition is similar.

The US DC (shown in Figure 8.1 and available at www.cdc.gov/nchs/data/dvs/death11-03final-acc.pdf) contains 3 basic sections that need completing by the **funeral director (FD)** and the **certifier (C)**. For comparison, the DC provided by the Ohio Department of Health/Vital Statistics is shown in Figure 8.2. The basic sections along with the individual responsible for its completion are:

1. Demographic and personal information of the deceased (FD)
2. Cause of Death (C)
3. Administrative (FD)

Each section contains sequentially numbered items and is accompanied by instructions on how to complete the referenced items. In addition to the cause-of-death section, certain items specifically pertain to the certifier and are important to complete. These include:

- Name of decedent (for deaths within a medical facility)
- Place of death (hospital or non-hospital)
- Facility name (medical, residence, moving vessel or vehicle)
- Location of death (city, county, state, zip code)
- Date and time or pronouncement of death
- Name, signature, and license number of pronouncing physician (when attending physician is unavailable)
- Actual or presumed date and time of death
- ME/C contact (Y/N)
- Cause of death
- Autopsy performance and availability of results upon certification (Y/N)
- Tobacco use
- Pregnancy status of females
- Manner of death
- Accident, injury or poison-related, date, time, place, location, and how injury occurred
- Work-related injury (Y/N)
- Transportation injury

The rationale behind this lengthy list of items is to capture key pieces of data including those that have direct bearing and influence on insurance pay-outs, those that facilitate gauging of the effectiveness of safety programs, and those that help to identify work-related hazards. Moreover, the charting of pregnancy status is the substrate for generating maternal mortality data. Furthermore, the accurate and succinct formulation of the cause-of-death statement that represents the decedent's one true lethal medical condition assures that the mortality data that is ultimately derived do not under- or over-represent a given disease category. Thus, it is important that the certifier complete all pertinent items.

The demographic and administrative sections are obtained by the FD from the **informant** who is usually the next-of-kin or a family member, the name of whom will be entered on the DC. With registering of a death, the FD has the responsibility to ensure that all of the sections are completed within the specified time as required by state law and to follow the instructions included on the death certificate regarding proper registration. The entering of the information into the sections can be done via a secure electronic format using the **electronic death registration system (EDRS)** operational in most states. A paper form of the DC can also be obtained from funeral homes, health departments, vital statistics agencies, and online for those without access to the electronic system. Certifiers that complete items manually, particularly the cause-of-death statement, must do so legibly as illegible entries will trigger notification by the vital statistics or health departments with request that the certifier revise any problematic or erroneous items, further delaying the certification and registration process. As of November of 2014, 41 states have an electronic death registration system for use by certifiers and funeral directors. Since the early 1900s, the collaborative efforts of members of the National Association for Public Health Statistics and Information Systems (NAPHSIS) have resulted in the continued optimization of vital statistics recording with emphasis on the secure and efficient exchange of vital records among jurisdictions with the EDRS as one result of those efforts [3]. With the timely provision death information needed by many for a variety of functions, the EDRS has greatly benefitted families, beneficiaries, insurance and financial institutions, funeral homes, and public health researchers.

There are two general phases necessary to complete a death certificate: **Certification** and **Registration**. These phases may take place one before or after the other or contemporaneously but must be done within a defined period of 5 days culminating into the official registration of the death with the state registrar. *Certification* involves the entering of not only the medical cause of death but also information about the death circumstances, other decedent conditions, and the manner of death. This is performed by the clinician certifier defined in the Introduction. It is necessary at this juncture to reiterate that **clinician certifiers certify natural deaths only and therefore only the 'natural' manner-of-death box is to be checked. Deaths suspected to have occurred as a result of accidental, suicidal, homicidal or suspicious circumstances or injury complications**

stemming from these should have already been or must promptly be reported to the ME/C. *Registration* involves the process of filing the death certificate at the city, county, and state level. The death certificate is ultimately filed with the state registrar's office by the funeral director in order for registration of the death to be official. In some states, the death certificate is a public record, available upon request and at cost.

A number of individuals and agencies are collectively involved in the certification, registration, and storage process of death certificates:

- Funeral Director (FD)
- Certifier of Death (C)
- Vital Statistics Office (VSO), Health Department (HD)
- State Registrar (SR)
- CDC-NCHS

The CDC-NCHS provides the **Model State Vital Statistics Act and Regulations** for the states to utilize as the basis for collection of death registration information [1]. It requires that a death be filed with the respective state VSO/HD within 5 days after the death. The FD of the funeral home chosen by the family will obtain identifying and demographic data from the next-of-kin or qualified informant within 48 hours of the death, and enter these data on the DC. The FD will then notify the C of the need to enter the medical cause of death on the DC. Upon notification, the C must enter the medical cause of death within 48 hours. If the death occurred in a medical institution, the authorized physician can begin the certification process by entering the decedent's name, date of death, medical cause of death, and electronic signature (or signature on paper form), all of which must be completed within 48 hours of the death. This partially completed DC allows the funeral home to remove the decedent from the medical facility and otherwise will then be made available to the FD for completion of the demographic and administrative sections through the EDRS system. If the cause of death is unavailable due to pending clinical test results or autopsy results, the certifier must indicate as such, for example by entering "Pending further study", "Pending autopsy results", or "Pending test results", or simply "Pending" in the Cause-of-Death Section within 48 hours of the death. Upon receipt and interpretation of clinical test or autopsy results, a supplemental death certificate (or a supplemental report to amend the original report of death) containing the etiologically specific medical cause of death must be completed within 5 days. If the death certificate has already been completed with the medical cause of death and additional medical information or autopsy results that would substantially change the cause of death have come to light, the original death certificate must be amended and the certifying physician must **immediately** notify the local or state VSO/HD to receive instructions on how to proceed.

Subsequent to completion of the requirements, registration of the DC can take place with the local and/or state VSO/HD and copies of death certificates can be obtained directly from local or county VSOs/HDs or via the FD. Completion of key designated requirements leading to death registration is also necessary in order for the FD to obtain authorization for final disposition by burial (burial permit) from the SR. Authorization for cremation (cremation permit) must be obtained from the ME/C or designated county official as prescribed by the SR.

The local VSO or HD will verify the accuracy and completeness of each DC and maintain a local copy prior to forwarding it to the SR. Incomplete or inaccurate information will require correction or revision by the FD or C, depending on which section is incomplete or inaccurate. Cause-of-death statements with wording describing injury or injury complications will be flagged and sent to the medical examiner/coroner in the corresponding jurisdiction. Cause-of-death statements that include non-specific disease conditions will also be flagged triggering a query process directed to the certifier of death in an effort to ensure that the most specific cause-of-death information is included. A list of more common medical diagnoses and conditions that are likely to be flagged appear in Chapter 3, Table 3.2. Finally, the SR will check the death certificate for accuracy and completeness and make queries as necessary and subsequently send compiled death data to the NCHS. The SR will also maintain record of the DC and serve as a source of certified copies and will also file the completed DC nationally with the CDC-NCHS. At every governmental level (city, county, state, and national) statistical data are compiled and analyzed for trends to facilitate decisions regarding preventative strategies and allocation of medical services and funding.

8.1.1 Registration of Fetal Deaths

The Model Vital Statistics Act requires that the death of a fetus be registered by reporting it to the State VSO or as otherwise directed by the SR within 5 days after delivery if the fetus weighs 350 grams or more or is of 20 weeks gestation or more. The identifying and demographic data must be obtained by the physician or representative of the medical institution. A fetal death with the above parameters occurring without medical attendance (i.e. spontaneous delivery at home) comes under the ME/C's jurisdiction and the respective office will investigate the death circumstances and will also certify the death. The death will subsequently be registered by reporting to the State within the required time period inclusive of the provision of amended reports as necessary and as required. A hospital fetal death with weight and gestational parameters below the limits specified above is processed as a surgical pathology specimen with gross anatomic and histological examination and issuance of a pathology report of findings and diagnoses, without issuance of a DC.

8.1.2 Nosology

Nosology is a branch of medicine that involves classification of disease. The medical cause of death as a single or sequela of disease and/or injury conditions appearing on the death certificate is reviewed and analyzed by mortality medical coders known as **nosologists** who are employed by the Division of Vital Statistics-NCHS. These are the trained professionals who utilize an extensive and detailed classification structure delineated in the International Classification of Diseases (ICD) and by application of established rules, derive alphanumeric ICD codes that define a particular disease or condition contained in hospital medical records or the *underlying cause of death* or *the other significant condition(s)* listed on the death certificate. Codes generated from DCs in turn are used to generate "single-cause mortality data" and "multiple-cause mortality data" [4]. As the disease (or injury) condition to occur earliest in the sequence leading to the death, the *underlying cause of death* is the main focus in coding as it represents the earliest in the chain of events where interventions and preventative measures would have the greatest impact on public health. Nosologists further ensure the accuracy of the coded data which facilitates the statistical derivation allowing the NCHS to release meaningful results by way of published reports and public-use data sets. *The more accurate and specific the disease (or injury) condition, the more accurate are the statistical and epidemiological data that are ultimately derived.* Listed below are a few examples of disease conditions referable to the heart, some of which are often used interchangeably as causes of death, but whose ICD codes differ by virtue of specificity or lack thereof:

- Cardiac arrest, unspecified-I46.9
- Sudden cardiac death-I46.1
- Cardiomyopathy-I42.9
- Acute transmural myocardial infarction of anterior wall-I21.0
- Hemopericardium following acute myocardial infarction-I23.0

The ICD coding system is published by the World Health Organization (WHO) and is currently in its 10th edition (ICD-10) with the 11th edition scheduled for release in 2018 [5]. The 11th edition will optimize comparison of mortality and clinical morbidity data in part through expansion of coding options. The ICD coding system is the international standard created for the reporting of diseases and health conditions and its flexible storage and retrieval formats allow analysis of health trends by researchers, health care providers, policy makers, and insurers. The US data is compiled with the mortality statistics from more than 70 countries for publication in the WHO's World Health Statistics annual report. This multipurpose report facilitates mortality studies relative to cause, location, demographics, and circumstances.

8.1.3 The Query Procedure and the Cause-of-Death Statement

The accuracy of ICD-coding by nosologists is directly related to the accuracy and completeness of the cause-of-death statement entered by the certifier of death. Thus, greater specificity and accuracy of the cause-of-death statement directly translates into more precise categorization and subcategorization of disease conditions that cause mortality and therefore more accurate mortality statistical information [6]. Inaccurate, vague, or incomplete statements may trigger a query procedure directed to the original certifier of the death, in an ultimate effort to maximize the accuracy of the final ICD-coding step [6]. The query procedure will require additional time and effort on the part of the certifier to respond to any deficiencies identified. Queries along with subsequent notification to the certifier are conducted by and will generally originate from the state vital statistics or registrar offices. The frequency and degree of querying varies by state due to variation in staffing numbers and fiscal support.

Based on the characteristics of the deficiency(ies) contained in the cause-of-death statement, the query will be assigned a priority level. A given priority level will cause a specific type of **query letter** to be generated. The query letter is addressed to the original certifier of the death and contains decedent information, the original cause-of-death statement, and requests for clarification or completion of deficient information. Six priority levels have been defined [7]:

- Level 1: queries to eliminate assumption based on inclusion of incomplete disease characteristics or use of non-specific terminology; ex. omission of histologic type (sarcoma vs carcinoma) of a malignant soft tissue tumor

- Level 2: queries for the clarification of non-specific conditions listed as the underlying cause of death; ex. listing myocardial rupture as the underlying cause of death which lacks etiologic specifics

- Level 3: queries requesting additional detail to allow classification of the underlying cause of death to a more specific disease category; ex. listing chronic liver disease as the underlying cause of death without inclusion of type (alcoholic cirrhosis, biliary cirrhosis, or cirrhosis due to chronic Hepatitis C infection)

- Level 4: queries requesting designation of specific organ or organ system; ex. listing embolism as the underlying cause of death with omission of the site and source

- Level 5: queries requesting additional information to assist in more precise subcategorization which is especially useful for researchers; ex. listing carcinomatosis due to carcinoid tumor of the small bowel with omission of the specific site of origin (such as terminal ileum)

- Level 6: the most thorough of the level of querying used to obtain specific terminology in order to eliminate any assumption even though such assumptions would likely be correct; ex. requiring specification that a cause of death listed as tuberculosis is in fact pulmonary tuberculosis

The query procedure can be beneficial for certifiers as it additionally serves as a training tool and is an effective method for acquainting or re-acquainting certifiers with the proper way of formulating a cause-of-death statement. They will be reminded of certain errors to be avoided when formulating the cause-of-death statement as these errors will likely trigger a query letter which will require valuable time and effort to address. Generally, these types of errors include: listing conditions in the incorrect order, citing non-specific conditions, listing conditions that lack a medical cause-and-effect relationship, entering of incorrect or illogical time intervals, omission of descriptive characteristics of malignancies and infections, and use of injury-associated terminology with omission of specifics of the injury or how the injury occurred. Peri-procedural deaths, which may either stem from the usual treatment of a natural disease or a therapeutic misadventure, needs clarification by the certifier in the requisite sections of the death certificate with inclusion of comprehensive and relevant terminology in the cause-of-death statement as this has direct bearing on ICD-coding by the nosologists. Peri-procedural death certification is further discussed in section 8.5.

8.2 Prerequisites for Signing the Death Certificate

The clinician certifier will certify a death in 2 basic instances: a natural death that was not reportable to the ME/C or a death that was reported to the ME/C but the ME/C opted not to take jurisdiction as the death circumstances and the history did not warrant assumption of such (i.e. a report and release death). Such report and released cases may have been reported due to a history of injury but the injury was so remote and without any documented clinicopathologic sequelae or resulted in only limited sequelae not medically linked with the death. The injury may have been more recent and associated with the terminal death circumstance, such as that acquired in a fall precipitated by sudden decompensation of chronic natural disease, but insufficient in extent and severity to constitute a cause or contributing factor in the death. A fall with head impact causing a lacerated scalp contusion precipitated by a hypertensive intracerebral hemorrhage confirmed clinically is one example of a non-jurisdictional death that is certifiable by the clinical practitioner. This is a typical scenario whereby it is presumed that the fall with head impact caused the intracerebral hemorrhage despite the fact that there may be clinical evidence to the contrary (i.e. history of poorly controlled hypertension, sphygmomanometric evidence of hypertension, or a hypertensive pattern of hemorrhage on neuroimaging).

Injury, such as limited bruising, abrasions, lacerations and non-debilitating fractures (i.e. nasal, phalangeal, wrist bones) sustained a short time prior to death may be evident but insufficient in severity to exacerbate underlying chronic natural disease. The "but for" principle is thus applicable, that *but for* the presence of minor (non-lethal) accidental injury, in the setting of natural disease with lethal potential, the patient would have died around the same time as when the injury was sustained.

A death occurring in the home or otherwise outside the confines of a medical facility in a decedent who has received medical evaluation and treatment for natural disease of known lethal potential within the preceding 12 months, whereby the death investigator for the ME/C (or police) has determined that there are no signs of foul play or significant trauma at the death scene, is certifiable by the clinician. Often, clinicians are reluctant to certify such deaths due to uncertainty regarding the cause of death or assumption that they are not obligated to certify a death that they did not physically attend. Moreover, *in-hospital* deaths, in which the patient dies of natural disease sequela subsequent to several hours of hospitalization, whereby medical records and diagnostic test results would be readily accessible for review and interpretation, are certifiable by the clinician regardless of the fact that the patient had not been evaluated within the preceding 12 months.

In summary, **the certifiable death for the clinician is one that has occurred expectedly or unexpectedly, even with minor injury, even if not in a medical facility, as a result of the process of natural disease or the aging process**. Once it has been determined that the death occurred naturally and is otherwise deemed not an ME/C case and before the certification process can continue, the certifier must:

- ✓ Be familiar with the state laws defining who is authorized and qualified to certify the death.
- ✓ Review the decedent's medical conditions and diagnoses noting the reason for the admission and if applicable, review the autopsy report and/or confer with the autopsy pathologist (facilitates identification of the underlying cause of death and completion of the expiration summary).
- ✓ If the death occurred at home, review the decedent's medical conditions and diagnoses and identify the entities with lethal potential (facilitates identification of underlying cause of death).

- ✓ Review concepts and definitions of cause, mechanism, and manner of death.
- ✓ Be familiar with the death certificate format and the certification process used in your state and the role of the Funeral Director in the registration process.

Information regarding death certification appearing in this chapter and preceding chapters is instructive and comprehensive. The 2003 revision of the *Physicians' Handbook on Medical Certification of Death*, published by the CDC is available online and is an additional, valuable resource for death certification instruction [8]. *The Cause of Death and the Death Certificate* is yet another useful and practical publication and product of the collaborative efforts of those directly involved in death certification [9].

8.3 Cause-of-Death Section: Structure and Definitions

The goal in creating a meaningful medical cause-of-death statement is to capture the essence of the events stemming from a single disease entity, listed in sequential fashion, that led to the patient's demise. If handwritten, legibility is an absolute requirement to better assist the tasks of the vital statistical and health department professionals in the registration process. If submitted electronically, the certifier is limited by a pre-defined number of character spaces within which to convey the essential cause-of-death components. The certifier must refrain from use of unestablished wording that is accusatory, admonishing, or that contains political or religious inference. For example, certain religious beliefs do not permit the transfusion of blood; thus, if a patient dies from a hematologic condition despite the use of blood substitutes in part as a result of refusal of conventional blood on religious grounds, the cause of death should not include any reference to the religious refusal. In this example, the medical cause of death is the hematological condition and related sequela. Furthermore, it is unnecessary to include wordage such as "medication non-compliance" or similar wording as it places blame on the decedent. Established terminology that at first glance may seem accusatory or admonishing such as "co-sleeping", "bed-sharing", "intravenous drug abuse", or "substance use disorder", are often included on death certificates generated by ME/C offices in order to flag specific historical and death scene attributes or high-risk behaviors associated with untimely death.

Inclusion of this type of terminology is essential for epidemiological study and monitoring of death trends.

The creation of a meaningful and concise cause-of-death statement is not only for coding purposes, but also to give future readers a general understanding of the medical cause of the individual's death without first having to access other records or to contact the certifying physician. The certifying physician must still be prepared to explain the meaning and context of the medical terminology used which will be unfamiliar to those without a medical background.

Before commencing to formulate the cause-of-death statement, one must have a working knowledge of the associated terminology. Some of the terms have been introduced and defined in previous chapters:

- **Cause-of-death statement**: the actual wording that constitutes the cause of the decedent's death; contains the underlying, immediate, and intermediate cause of death and may contain one or more other significant conditions
- **Underlying cause of death**: the etiologically specific disease or injury condition that precipitated a series of medical events that ultimately led to the death; temporally, the most remote
- **Immediate cause of death**: the final disease or injury condition that resulted from the underlying cause death; temporally, occurring closest to the time of death
- **Intermediate cause of death**: the disease or injury condition that resulted from the underlying cause of death and medically linked to and occurring prior to the immediate cause of death; temporally occurring between the underlying and the immediate cause of death
- **Mechanism of death**: the non-specific physiological derangement or biochemical disturbance of function that is triggered by the underlying cause of death or simply the means by which the underlying cause of death exerts its lethal effect; sometimes a component of the intermediate or immediate cause of death but never to be used as an underlying cause of death (ex. hepatic encephalopathy)
- **Non-specific (anatomic) process**: a non-specific macroscopic or microscopic change that is triggered by a more specific disease entity or entities including the underlying disease entity; can cause physiologic derangement and thus represents a conduit of the mechanism of death (ex. hepatic

cirrhosis is the anatomic process that can cause the derangement hepatic encephalopathy)

- **Other significant condition**: pre-existing or co-existing conditions that contribute to the death but do not result in the underlying cause of death; includes risk factors or simply other contributing conditions
- **Manner of death**: classification of death based on the circumstances that led to it or simply the way in which the death came to be; i.e natural, accident, suicide, homicide, and undetermined; clinicians certify only natural deaths thus would select or enter only the natural manner-of-death classification

After reviewing the pertinent terminology, familiarity with the basic structure of the pertinent section of the death certificate is in order. For the sake of brevity, other items such as pregnancy status, tobacco use, injury information, and autopsy information have been omitted. Explanation regarding those items is provided in the instructions that accompany every death certificate. The cause-of-death section, depicted below, consists of 4 main sections: Part I, Part II, a section for listing the interval of time between the onset and death, and the manner-of-death section. Part I is for the main cause-of-death statement, with up to 4 lines that can be utilized; Part II is for listing one or more significant contributing conditions. Below is the basic structure and format of the cause-of-death section taken from the US Standard Certificate of Death:

<table>
<tr><td>Part I.

A.</td><td>Approximate interval: Onset to death</td></tr>
<tr><td>Due to (or as a consequence of):
B.</td><td></td></tr>
<tr><td>Due to (or as a consequence of):
C.</td><td></td></tr>
<tr><td>Due to (or as a consequence of):
D.</td><td></td></tr>
<tr><td colspan="2">Part II. Other significant conditions contributing to death but not resulting in the underlying cause given in Part I</td></tr>
<tr><td></td><td>Manner of Death</td></tr>
</table>

Each line in Part I is designated for a particular component of the cause-of-death statement as defined previously:

Part I. A. **Immediate cause of death**	Approximate interval: Onset to death
Due to (or as a consequence of): B. **Intermediate cause of death**	
Due to (or as a consequence of): C. **Intermediate cause of death**	
Due to (or as a consequence of): D. **Underlying cause of death**	
Part II. Other significant conditions contributing to death but not resulting in the underlying cause given in Part I	
	Manner of Death

The ordering of the lines in Part I reflects the sequence of the developing disease conditions or its complications starting with the most recent component (the immediate cause of death) which occupies line A, to the intervening components which occupy lines B and C (the intermediate cause of death), to the component occurring farthest back in time and which occupies line D (the underlying cause of death). **The underlying cause of death is the most important part of the cause-of-death statement, must have etiologic specificity, and must always be included.** ICD coding, discussed in section 8.1, is based largely on the underlying cause-of-death information.

There must be a sequential, medically understood, cause-and-effect relationship between the components listed on each line. Simplistically, if read out aloud: “A is due to or as a consequence of B, which is due to or as a consequence of C, which is due to or as a consequence of D. Or using a realistic example: “Hemopericardium with cardiac tamponade is due to or as a consequence of acute myocardial infarct with spontaneous ventricular rupture, which is due to or as a consequence of coronary arterial thrombosis, which is due to or as a consequence of atherosclerotic coronary artery disease”. As entered in the cause-of-death section with inclusion of time intervals and manner-of-death classification, the realistic example appears as:

Part I.	Approximate interval: Onset to death
A. **Hemopericardium with cardiac tamponade**	**Hours**
Due to (or as a consequence of): B. **Acute myocardial infarct with spontaneous ventricular rupture**	**5 days**
Due to (or as a consequence of): C. **Coronary arterial thrombosis**	**7 Days**
Due to (or as a consequence of): D. **Atherosclerotic coronary artery disease**	**Decades**
Part II. Other significant conditions contributing to death but not resulting in the underlying cause given in Part I	
	Manner of Death **Natural**

In the above example, while a quasi-specific, physiologic derangement is listed as the immediate cause of death, its occurrence is explained by the provision of the intermediate conditions, and most importantly the underlying disease condition that ultimately led to it.

It is important to enter the **time interval** in the designated box next to *each* line item in Part I based on the patient's available medical information, to the best of the clinician's knowledge. Verification of the presence chronic disease conditions may be important for research and insurance purposes. Use of terms such as seconds, minutes, hours, days, weeks, years, and decades with or without specific numbers are permitted. Use of qualifying terms such as "approximately" or "unknown" is also permitted. If the time of onset to death is not known, then "unknown" must be entered. It is not optional and otherwise is not permissible to leave the time interval boxes blank.

Pre-existing or co-existing conditions present at the time of death but otherwise well-controlled, without recent exacerbation, and not connected with the sequence of events in Part I, can be listed in Part II. These conditions are often relevant to what appears in Part I and gives a more complete picture of the decedent's overall health status at the time of death. These are disease conditions primarily but can include environmental, behavioral or demographic risk factors such as obesity, oral contraception use, depression, excessive environmental heat or cold, tobacco smoking, and substance use disorder. Like other items on the DC form, entities listed in Part II provide data utilized in epidemiological studies. Hypertension with clinically or anatomically evident cardiac disease often co-exists with atherosclerotic cardiovascular disease, and in the appropriate clinical context, could qualify as another significant condition as the co-existence of this disease would be an additional compromising health component although not opined to be the cause of death:

Part I.	Approximate interval: Onset to death
A. **Hemopericardium with cardiac tamponade**	**Hours**
Due to (or as a consequence of): B. **Acute myocardial infarct with spontaneous ventricular rupture**	**5 days**
Due to (or as a consequence of): C. **Coronary arterial thrombosis**	**7 Days**
Due to (or as a consequence of): D. **Atherosclerotic coronary artery disease**	**Decades**
Part II. Other significant conditions contributing to death but not resulting in the underlying cause given in Part I **Hypertensive cardiovascular disease**	
	Manner of Death **Natural**

It is not necessary to use all of the lines in Part I, thus from 1 up to 4 lines may be used and the lowermost line always represents the underlying cause of death and must be etiologically specific. This is illustrated in the following examples:

For a scenario that includes a history of hyperlipidemia, and clinical and imaging evidence of a myocardial infarct with fluid in the pericardial cavity, angiographic evidence of coronary arterial stenosis, but without a diagnosis of coronary arterial thrombosis the statement may be formulated as:

Part I.	Approximate interval: Onset to death
A. **Hemopericardium with cardiac tamponade**	**Hours**
Due to (or as a consequence of): B. **Acute myocardial infarct with spontaneous ventricular rupture**	**3 Days**
Due to (or as a consequence of): C. **Atherosclerotic cardiovascular disease**	**Decades**
Due to (or as a consequence of): D.	
Part II. Other significant conditions contributing to death but not resulting in the underlying cause given in Part I	
	Manner of Death **Natural**

For a scenario with a history of hyperlipidemia, recent history of chest pain, clinical evidence of a myocardial infarct and angiographic/imaging evidence of coronary artery disease the statement may be formulated as:

Part I.	Approximate interval: Onset to death
A. **Acute myocardial infarct**	**Days**
Due to (or as a consequence of): B. **Atherosclerotic coronary artery disease**	**Decades**
Due to (or as a consequence of): C.	
Due to (or as a consequence of): D.	
Part II. Other significant conditions contributing to death but not resulting in the underlying cause given in Part I	
	Manner of Death **Natural**

If known, inclusion of the affected coronary artery can be done as well (i.e. "Atherosclerotic coronary artery disease, left anterior descending coronary artery"). In the above scenario, arrhythmia would be the likely mechanism of death and also may have been captured electrocardiographically. It is not necessary to include mechanisms, however. Inclusion of mechanisms is not prohibited, but they must be accompanied by the etiologically specific entity that led to it.

For a scenario of a sudden death occurring at home without death scene findings of foul play or trauma by the medicolegal death investigator, with a history of hyperlipidemia with moderate 3-vessel coronary artery stenosis found on angiography 2 years prior to death, and with a recent history of worsening chest pain and shortness of breath, the statement may be formulated as:

Part I. A. **Atherosclerotic coronary artery disease**	Approximate interval: Onset to death **Decades**
Due to (or as a consequence of): B.	
Due to (or as a consequence of): C.	
Due to (or as a consequence of): D.	
Part II. Other significant conditions contributing to death but not resulting in the underlying cause given in Part I	
	Manner of Death **Natural**

An acute change in plaque morphology with plaque rupture and luminal thrombosis of a coronary artery, coronary artery vasospasm, an acute myocardial infarct, or arrhythmia are all medically known complications of coronary artery disease. Furthermore, given the historical information in this scenario, a sudden cardiac death is a reasonable assumption. The cause-of-death statement is one of probability, that more likely than not or with more than 50% certainty, given known clinical and historical information, the certifier *opines* that the cause of death is as entered. It is permissible then to indicate uncertainty in a cause-of-death statement. Using the same scenario above the statement may be formulated as:

Part I.	Approximate interval: Onset to death
A. **Probable acute myocardial infarct with sudden cardiac death**	**Days**
Due to (or as a consequence of): B. **Atherosclerotic coronary artery disease**	**Decades**
Due to (or as a consequence of): C.	
Due to (or as a consequence of): D.	
Part II. Other significant conditions contributing to death but not resulting in the underlying cause given in Part I	
	Manner of Death **Natural**

With a history of hyperlipidemia, recent history of chest pain, and ventricular fibrillation captured electrocardiographically by medical first responders, a reasonable statement that indicates uncertainty may be formulated as:

Part I.	Approximate interval: Onset to death
A. **Ventricular-fibrillation arrest with sudden cardiac death**	**Minutes**
Due to (or as a consequence of): B. **Probable atherosclerotic cardiovascular disease**	**Decades**
Due to (or as a consequence of): C.	
Due to (or as a consequence of): D.	
Part II. Other significant conditions contributing to death but not resulting in the underlying cause given in Part I	
	Manner of Death Natural

In certain circumstances of natural death whereby the death occurred prior to *any* clinical workup, prior to a *complete* clinical workup or that occurred after a complete workup that yielded insufficient, uninterpretable or non-specific diagnostic information, use of qualifying words and phrases may be necessary. In other circumstances, there may be little or no clinical history or a non-specific clinical presentation. Qualifying words and phrases include:

- presumed or probable
- unknown or uncertain cause
- etiology or cause undetermined
- etiology or cause uncertain
- undetermined natural cause
- type undetermined or unspecified
- type not otherwise specified

Use of such words and phrases is permissible but should be done only after all efforts have been made to determine the cause of death inclusive of performance of an autopsy.

For a scenario of a sudden death in a chronic alcoholic with longstanding hepatic cirrhosis presenting with sudden massive hematemesis following a bout of coughing the cause-of-death statement may be formulated as:

Part I.	Approximate interval: Onset to death
A. **Spontaneous acute upper gastrointestinal hemorrhage**	**Minutes**
Due to (or as a consequence of): B. **Probable (or Presumed) Ruptured esophageal varix**	**Hours**
Due to (or as a consequence of): C. **Clinicopathologic sequela of hepatic cirrhosis**	**Years**
Due to (or as a consequence of): D. **Chronic alcoholism**	**Years**
Part II. Other significant conditions contributing to death but not resulting in the underlying cause given in Part I	
	Manner of Death **Natural**

Based on the information in the above scenario, it is reasonable to opine that the prolonged cirrhotic state in all probability led to portal hypertension (a sequela) which in turn led to the formation of esophageal varices and spontaneous rupture exacerbated by coughing. Use of the qualifying words also indicates that a definitive clinical diagnosis was not or could not be made. Inclusion of the word "spontaneous" is important as it specifies that the hemorrhaging was not associated with trauma.

For a scenario of a death following sudden massive hematemesis with a history of chronic non-steroidal anti-inflammatory use and recent abrupt onset of stomach pain, peptic ulcer disease rises to the top of the differential of potential causes but absent a definitive clinical diagnosis, the inclusion of qualifying terminology is in order. The cause-of-death statement in this case may be formulated as:

Part I. A. **Spontaneous acute upper gastrointestinal hemorrhage**	Approximate interval: Onset to death **Minutes**
Due to (or as a consequence of): B. **Probable (or Presumed) peptic ulcer disease**	**Months** **(or Years)**
Due to (or as a consequence of): C.	
Due to (or as a consequence of): D.	
Part II. Other significant conditions contributing to death but not resulting in the underlying cause given in Part I	
	Manner of Death **Natural**

It may be necessary to include qualifying terminology with a non-specific process in light of little supportive medical history and without an autopsy to provide a specific etiology, such as in a scenario of massive hematemesis lacking historical information. In that case, the cause-of-death statement may be formulated as:

Part I.	Approximate interval: Onset to death
A. **Spontaneous acute upper gastrointestinal hemorrhage**	**Minutes**
Due to (or as a consequence of): B. **Undetermined natural cause (s)**	**Unknown**
Due to (or as a consequence of): C.	
Due to (or as a consequence of): D.	
Part II. Other significant conditions contributing to death but not resulting in the underlying cause given in Part I	
	Manner of Death **Natural**

For a scenario of an elderly female found dead in bed within her secured residence without significant medical history or recent medical complaints, with regular annual physical examinations by a primary care physician, and with no signs of foul play, trauma, or intoxicants found at the death scene, using the qualifying terminology, the cause-of-death statement may be formulated as:

Part I.	Approximate interval: Onset to death
A. **Undetermined natural cause(s)**	**Unknown**
Due to (or as a consequence of): B.	
Due to (or as a consequence of): C.	
Due to (or as a consequence of): D.	
Part II. Other significant conditions contributing to death but not resulting in the underlying cause given in Part I	
	Manner of Death **Natural**

In this scenario, the approximate time interval is also unknown and is listed as such. In this scenario, the same cause-of-death statement would apply had an autopsy been performed to find a heart of normal weight and configuration, mild atherosclerotic coronary artery stenosis, and negative or non-contributory findings on toxicological and chemistry testing. The use of qualifying terminology in this instance emphasizes the natural death circumstances while at the same time acknowledges the clinical diagnostic limitations in determining the precise cause in a sudden death occurring outside the confines of a medical facility. Moreover, while an autopsy with postmortem analysis of bodily fluids can provide a cause of death in many instances and exclude other causes as well, it too has limitations, particularly as it relates to sudden neurological and cardiac deaths without demonstrable pathology.

8.4 Death Certificate Errors

It is conceivable that uncertainty regarding the whole death certification process arises out of the brevity and infrequency of instruction on how to formulate the cause-of-death statement, beginning with the first year of residency. A number of remedies can help to dispel this uncertainty including tutorials given by forensic pathologists and officials from health departments and state registrar offices, in-service exercises for resident and attending physician staff, and in-service examinations for residents with follow-up and feedback on performance. Moreover, regularly scheduled review of death certificates completed by physicians with clinical correlation by a mortality review committee can be done and should require participation by residents at all levels of training, particularly those training in the primary care specialties.

Unfortunately, the uncertainty regarding death certification has persisted and given rise to erroneous and incomplete death certificates which have direct effects on the time-sensitive registration and mortality data compilation processes. As explained in the 8.1 subsection, erroneous and incomplete death certificates will trigger a query process in which the certifier is notified of missing and/or incomplete information and must expend an additional period of valuable time to address the query. Furthermore, erroneous or incomplete cause-of-death statements affect the accuracy of coding performed by nosologists. Errors on death certificates are problematic not only because they misrepresent the decedent's true cause-of-death circumstances but also create problems and lead to delays regarding settlement of estate matters, insurance payouts, death registration, and vital statistics calculations. Problems and delays arise not only from erroneous cause-of-death-statements but also from incomplete or skipped items and therefore it is important to follow the instructions included with the death certificate and to complete all relevant items.

A clear understanding of the significance of each one of the patient's medical conditions and their lethal potential within the context of the terminal clinical course is a prerequisite for accurate cause-of-death determination. Incomplete or misinterpreted clinical information can lead to errors in conclusion as to what led to the patient's demise. Errors in clinical conclusion, including conclusions found on death certificates, have been demonstrated in studies comparing clinical diagnoses to autopsy findings, again proving the value of the autopsy [10,11].

Previous studies have analyzed and tabulated the different types of errors on death certificates in order to help improve the accuracy of death certification by clinicians [12,13,14]. Below is a list of errors to be avoided when formulating Part I and Part II of the death certificate and is representative of those highlighted in previous studies and based on the author's own experience with the review and evaluation of numerous erroneous death certificates. Following the list and corresponding to each item on the list are example cause-of-death statements, with time intervals intentionally left blank in most cases:

- Incorrect sequencing or reversal of order of statements
- Use of abbreviations and shorthand
- Listing of more than one competing disease or disease conditions per line
- Sequential listing of causally unrelated disease or disease conditions
- Citing of mechanisms, terminal events, or non-specific processes with omission of the specific etiology or etiologic agent (ex. ventricular fibrillation, cardiac/respiratory arrest, cardiac/respiratory failure, asystole, organ failure, sepsis, etc.)
- Omission of descriptive characteristics of malignancies (site, cell type, grade, stage, right versus left side)
- Inclusion of injury or injury-related complication in Part I OR Part II with selection of "natural" manner-of-death classification
- Reversal of Part I or Part II cause-of-death information

Incorrect sequencing/reversal of order:

Part I.	Approximate interval: Onset to death
A. **Atherosclerotic coronary artery disease**	**Years**
Due to (or as a consequence of): B. **Acute myocardial infarct**	**7 Days**
Due to (or as a consequence of): C. **Spontaneous acute myocardial rupture**	**Hours**
Due to (or as a consequence of): D. **Hemopericardium with cardiac tamponade**	**Minutes**
Part II. Other significant conditions contributing to death but not resulting in the underlying cause given in Part I	

In the above example, hemopericardium with cardiac tamponade is the *end result* of a ruptured myocardial infarct caused by atherosclerotic coronary artery disease, not the start of the chain of events and therefore should not be listed on line D as it is not the underlying cause of death. Atherosclerotic coronary artery disease however, is the longest standing disease condition and is medically known to cause myocardial infarction which over time can lead to rupture and subsequent hemopericardium with cardiac tamponade. Recognition that the time intervals should progressively *increase*, not decrease when read from top to bottom can help insure that the statements are listed correspondingly and in correct order.

Use of abbreviations and shorthand:

Part I.	Approximate interval: Onset to death
A. **PE**	
Due to (or as a consequence of): B. **DVT**	
Due to (or as a consequence of): C. **HCVD w/ CHF**	
Due to (or as a consequence of): D .	
Part II. Other significant conditions contributing to death but not resulting in the underlying cause given in Part I **NIDDM, HLD, CLD, PAD**	

Abbreviations and shorthand notations are potentially problematic for nosologists, researchers, and anyone else who reviews death certificates. There are a number of medical abbreviations that are commonly used in medical practice and are also recognized by nosologists, but it cannot be assumed with absolute certainty that the abbreviation(s) used correspond to the disease(s) intended by the certifier. The use of punctuation marks (other than commas and periods) and arithmetic symbols should also be avoided. In the example above, the disease conditions should be written out for the purpose of clarification as there may be multiple possible translations, some also with lethal potential, as described below:

- PE: pulmonary embolism or more precisely pulmonary thromboembolism or pulmonary arterial thromboembolism; also stands for pre-ecclampsia and physical examination
- DVT: deep venous thrombosis; the involved extremity should also be included if known, i.e. deep venous thrombosis of lower extremities, or right/left lower extremity
- HCVD w/ CHF: hypertensive cardiovascular disease with congestive heart failure; CHF also stands for congenital hepatic fibrosis and cyclophosphamide, hexamethylmelamine, 5-fluorouracil (cancer drug regimen)
- NIDDM: Non-Insulin Dependent Diabetes Mellitus

- HLD: hyperlipidemia; also stands for hypersensitivity lung disease, Hippel Lindau Disease, herniated lumbar disc
- CLD: chronic liver disease; also stands for chronic lung disease
- PAD: peripheral arterial disease; also stands for peripheral air-space disease, post-admission day, passive acquired anti-D

Listing more than one competing disease or disease condition per line:

Part I. A. **Coronary artery disease and pulmonary emphysema**	Approximate interval: Onset to death
Due to (or as a consequence of): B.	
Due to (or as a consequence of): C.	
Due to (or as a consequence of): D.	
Part II. Other significant conditions contributing to death but not resulting in the underlying cause given in Part I	

The worst of the 2 conditions should be selected, in keeping with the decedent's terminal course, recent signs and symptoms, clinical diagnostic information and application of the classification scheme for lethal disease potential presented at the end of Chapter 7. The other condition could reasonably be listed in Part II. Hypertensive cardiovascular disease and atherosclerotic cardiovascular disease are examples of 2 related, often co-existing and significant conditions where the temptation to list the cause of death as "Hypertensive atherosclerotic cardiovascular disease" may arise. At times, it may be difficult to decipher on clinical grounds, even with the addition of autopsy findings, which of the diseases was the start of the terminal chain of lethal events, whereby as a last resort, both of the diseases could be listed. However, if the clinical presentation and/or history of present illness indicate an acutely evolving myocardial ischemic process (history of hypercholesterolemia, chest pain following exertion, and EKG findings of ischemia), then a reasonable cause-of-death statement that ensures more accurate nosological coding would be:

Part I. A. **Atherosclerotic cardiovascular disease**	Approximate interval: Onset to death
Due to (or as a consequence of): B.	
Due to (or as a consequence of): C.	
Due to (or as a consequence of): D.	
Part II. Other significant conditions contributing to death but not resulting in the underlying cause given in Part I **Hypertensive cardiovascular disease**	

Sequential listing of causally unrelated diseases or disease conditions:

Part I. A. **Coronary artery disease**	Approximate interval: Onset to death **15 years**
Due to, or as a consequence of: B. **Pulmonary emphysema**	**10 years**
Due to, or as a consequence of: C. **Stage IV kidney disease**	**8 years**
Due to, or as a consequence of: D. **Hypertensive encephalopathy**	**1 week**
Part II. Other significant conditions contributing to death but not resulting in the underlying cause given in Part I	

There is no medically known, cause-and-effect relationship between coronary artery disease, pulmonary emphysema, Stage IV kidney disease, and hypertensive encephalopathy. This example is also representative of instances in which the certifier accesses the list of the patient's medical diagnoses and simply lists the top few in Part I without regard that there must be a sequential, medically known, cause-and-effect relationship between the disease conditions listed on the lines. The lines in Part I are not to be used as a "laundry list" for the haphazard listing of a few of the patient's medical conditions. Furthermore, recognition that the corresponding time intervals do not progressively increase when read from top to bottom also signifies the lack of causal relationship between the disease conditions and should prompt review of the most clinically prominent of the patient's medical conditions and revision of the cause-of-death statement with proper sequencing.

Citing mechanisms, terminal events, or a non-specific process (es) and conditions with omission of the specific etiology or etiologic agent. Two examples:

1.

Part I. A. **Cardiopulmonary arrest**	Approximate interval: Onset to death
Due to (or as a consequence of): B. **Congestive heart failure**	
Due to (or as a consequence of): C.	
Due to (or as a consequence of): D.	
Part II. Other significant conditions contributing to death but not resulting in the underlying cause given in Part I	

In this example, it is unknown what led to the congestive heart failure which is a mechanism of death that lacks specificity. Was it hypertensive cardiovascular disease, chronic obstructive pulmonary disease due to emphysema, or valvular heart disease due to calcific aortic stenosis? It is also unnecessary to list terminal events such as cardiopulmonary arrest which are common final pathways to the cessation to vital function. **It is never permissible to list terminal events as the underlying cause of death.** Other examples of terminal events are cardiac arrest, respiratory arrest, asystole, ventricular fibrillation, pulseless electrical activity, and electromechanical disassociation. It is permissible to list physiologic derangements or non-specific disease processes as intermediate and immediate causes for clarification purposes, **as long as they are accompanied by an etiologically specific disease condition medically known to be associated with it** (Refer to Table 7.1 for an expanded list). Inclusion of such derangements or processes helps researchers understand aspects of disease progression which can ultimately aid in reduction of morbidity and mortality through targeted clinical interventions. The physiologic derangement or process can be listed *with* the etiologic entity on the same line or on a separate line above it. If listed separately, the specific etiologic entity would then be listed below it or on the lowermost line where it is properly designated as the underlying cause of death (see first few examples in section 8.3). **Signs and symptoms** are also commonly non-specific as to a cause and usually evoke a differential list of potential diagnoses. Likewise, signs and symptoms should not be cited in the cause-of-death statement.

2.

Part I. A. **Meningitis with sepsis**	Approximate interval: Onset to death
Due to (or as a consequence of): B.	
Due to (or as a consequence of): C.	
Due to (or as a consequence of): D.	
Part II. Other significant conditions contributing to death but not resulting in the underlying cause given in Part I	

In this example, in addition to listing the non-specific term "sepsis", the causative agent is omitted leaving many unanswered questions. Was the meningitis caused by a bacterium or a virus? Was the sepsis bacterial, representing a secondary infection in the setting of viral meningitis? Was the organism responsible for the meningitis the same organism that caused the sepsis? Is this a polymicrobial infection? Does this represent transmitted/transmissible infection or opportunistic infection in a patient with acquired or genetically-based immunodeficiency? Does this represent an isolated infection or a part of a cluster of infections arising from a particular location or associated with a particular vector or other source? The answers to these questions could have widespread public health ramifications, both immediate and delayed. Moreover, there are federal, state, and local mandates requiring the timely reporting of certain infectious diseases. Oversight with data collection, compilation, and reporting is performed by the National Notifiable Diseases Surveillance System (NNDSS), an arm of the CDC [15].

Omission of descriptive characteristics of malignancy:

Part I. A. **Metastatic cancer**	Approximate interval: Onset to death
Due to (or as a consequence of): B.	
Due to (or as a consequence of): C.	
Due to (or as a consequence of): D.	
Part II. Other significant conditions contributing to death but not resulting in the underlying cause given in Part I	

In this example, the type, stage, grade and primary site (or origin) are omitted. These specifics can be obtained from surgical, cytological, or autopsy pathology reports. Examples of *type* include adenocarcinoma, squamous cell carcinoma, sarcoma, leukemia, and lymphoma. *Stages* 1-4 are included to indicate extent of spread of the disease. Poorly-, moderately-, or well-differentiated terms define *grade*. The organ from which the cancer originated, or the *site* should be included (ie brain, breast, prostate gland, colon, liver, bone, etc.). Where applicable or when known, the anatomic side of location (right or left) should be included. It is acknowledged that at times information regarding site, stage, grade, and origin may be unknown, unobtainable, or an autopsy was not performed. Inclusion of qualifying terminology such as "Metastatic cancer of unknown origin, type, and grade" may be necessary. As an example, an all-inclusive cause-of-death statement for a malignancy could be written as: "Stage IV moderately-differentiated invasive ductal adenocarcinoma of the right breast".

Inclusion of injury or injury-related complication in Part I or II while manner of death marked as "natural" (2 examples follow):

1.

Part I.	Approximate interval: Onset to death
A. **Urosepsis**	
Due to (or as a consequence of): B. **Chronic polymicrobial urinary tract infection**	
Due to (or as a consequence of): C. **Urogenic bladder with chronic catheterization**	
Due to (or as a consequence of): D. **Remote thoracic spinal cord injury with paraplegia**	
Part II. Other significant conditions contributing to death but not resulting in the underlying cause given in Part I	
	Manner of Death **Natural**

2.

Part I.	Approximate interval: Onset to death
A. **Spontaneous acute intracerebral hemorrhage**	
Due to (or as a consequence of): B. **Hypertensive cerebrovascular disease**	
Due to (or as a consequence of): C.	
Due to (or as a consequence of): D.	
Part II. Other significant conditions contributing to death but not resulting in the underlying cause given in Part I **Remote thoracic spinal cord injury with paraplegia**	
	Manner of Death **Natural**

Whenever injury (or injury complication) is a cause or contributing factor in the death, **regardless of the time interval between the injury and the onset of the complication**, the manner of death can no longer be considered as natural even when the immediate or intermediate entities are recognized as natural disease conditions. One or more pathophysiological explanations are possible in the setting of injury as a cause or contributing factor such as catecholamine-mediated cardiovascular effects, hemorrhage, infection with systemic inflammatory complications, soft tissue swelling with vascular compromise, cerebral edema with herniation, and the many sequelae of immobility. As illustrated in the cause-of-death examples above, paraplegia can lead to chronic urinary tract infection with urosepsis but if paraplegia was caused by a traumatic injury, then the manner of death is not purely a natural one. Traumatic spinal cord injury of the mid-thoracic level can give rise to autonomic dysreflexia and cause uncontrolled hypertension with the risk of spontaneous hypertensive intracerebral hemorrhage. Intracerebral hemorrhage may also be associated with pre-existing or co-existing primary hypertensive cardio- and cerebrovascular disease.

The presence of injury or injury-associated complications (or intoxication and intoxication-associated complications), whether as part of the cause-of-death chain of events or as a contributing (Part II) condition, has bearing on the manner-of-death classification which is dependent upon the circumstances surrounding the death (i.e. accidental, homicidal, or suicidal). A rule-of-thumb to help remember this important point is: **"trauma (or intoxication) trumps natural manner of death"** The unqualified use of words like "accident" such as in cerebrovascular accident, "injury" such as in acute kidney injury or anoxic brain injury, and "fracture" should also be avoided due to manner-of-death implications. Phraseology such as "spontaneous acute intracerebral hemorrhage due to essential hypertension" is preferable to "cerebral vascular accident" in order to specify the non-traumatic origin of the brain pathology. Similarly, use of the term "encephalopathy" rather than "brain injury" or the terms "kidney/renal ischemia" rather than "kidney/renal injury" are preferable as long as they are accompanied by the etiologically specific entity. With use of the word *fracture*, it must be ascertained as to whether it is pathological or traumatic in origin. Deaths arising from *pathological* fractures resulting from disease conditions such as osteoporosis or metastatic cancer are representative of the sequela of natural disease processes and can be correctly classified as natural in manner. However at times, a fall or some other type of blunt force trauma causes a fracture in an individual with bone that is already compromised by natural disease. In that instance, if the fracture is considered to be a cause or contributing factor in the death, then the manner of death must be a classified as something other than natural, based on the circumstances that led to the fracture, most commonly accidental, which falls under the purview of the ME/C. At other times, there is uncertainty as to whether trauma was the cause of the fracture or it could not be verified clinically. **Deaths known or suspected to be associated with injury/injury complications or intoxicant/intoxicant complications must be reported to the ME/C for further investigation and the clinician is absolved from completion of the death certificate, once jurisdiction has been taken.**

Reversal of Part I and II cause-of-death information:

Part I. A. **Diabetes Mellitus**	Approximate interval: Onset to death
Due to (or as a consequence of): B.	
Due to (or as a consequence of): C.	
Due to (or as a consequence of): D.	
Part II. Other significant conditions contributing to death but not resulting in the underlying cause given in Part I **Hemopericardium, spontaneous rupture of acute myocardial infarct, atherosclerotic coronary artery disease with plaque rupture and luminal thrombosis**	

In this example, the overriding chain of events, temporally closest to the death is the ruptured myocardial infarct with hemopericardium caused by the thrombosed coronary artery affected by atherosclerosis. These chain of events should be listed sequentially in Part I and would be read as "*Hemopericardium due to spontaneous rupture of acute myocardial infarct due to coronary arterial thrombosis due to atherosclerotic coronary artery disease*". Diabetes Mellitus is recognized as a cause of death by a number of mechanisms including metabolic derangement and effects on multiple organs. It also often co-exists in patients with atherosclerotic cardiovascular disease. However, a patient with well-controlled diabetes may also die *with* rather that from the disease which is also known to promote atherogenesis and the development of atherosclerosis, but not directly cause it. Thus, in this example, Diabetes Mellitus should be listed in Part II as it contributed to but is not a direct cause of the events stemming directly from atherosclerotic coronary artery disease.

8.5 Peri-procedural and Therapy-Associated Death Certification

Deaths suspected or known to be a complication of the application of diagnostic, therapeutic, surgical or anesthetic interventions are reportable in many jurisdictions. ME/C offices have investigated and continue to investigate these types of deaths inclusive of autopsy performance, review of medical records, and consultation with clinicians with expertise pertinent to the medical intervention of concern [16]. The proper certification of these deaths is essential as the information contained on the death certificates can help illuminate problems regarding treatment modalities, diagnostic procedures, medications, and medical devices that may be linked to untoward morbidity and mortality. Issues regarding deviation from standards of care, incorrect use of medical devices, or administration of the incorrect type and amount of medication may also be illuminated along with the potential to trigger litigation. Clinicians who do certify these deaths (*or any death*) must be objective and forthright in the formulation of the cause-of-death statement and resist the inclination to mute or conceal the true cause of death whether out of concern for causing upset to the family or out of concern that litigation may follow. When there is uncertainty regarding proper cause and manner-of-death determination of peri-procedural deaths, reporting the death to the ME/C and/or direct consultation with a forensic pathologist is in order. The monitoring of peri-procedural deaths is an important facet in the monitoring and maintenance of public health.

The manner-of-death determination in peri-procedural deaths will depend upon the surrounding circumstances, particularly the temporal relationship with the intervention and the ensuing complications, with accident, natural, or undetermined options more commonly used for classification. Variation amongst forensic pathologists regarding of manner-of-death classification in these types of deaths is a given and is based on practice experience and depth of knowledge of the vast number of medical procedures and interventions. If the extent and severity of the natural disease make death likely and imminent with or without therapeutic intervention, then the natural manner-of-death classification would be most appropriate. This logic utilizes the "but for" principle that but for the therapeutic intervention the patient *would* have died from the natural disease. Deaths occurring after emergency surgery for catastrophic natural disease qualify for natural manner-of-death classification.

Therapeutic complication is used in some ME/C jurisdictions as a classification of manner of death or as a variant of the natural manner-of-death classification, in order to highlight that a death was temporally associated with the administration of appropriate medical therapy or that occurred during the normal course of a diagnostic procedure to treat or diagnose natural disease. If *but for* the therapeutic intervention the patient would *not* have died or was not expected to die from the natural disease, then the designation of therapeutic complication would apply. Death occurring after elective surgery for a stable disease condition would be a general example. The classification of a death as a therapeutic complication does not imply that negligence or some degree of malpractice occurred but rather brings to the attention that certain medical therapies and procedures used to treat natural disease carry a risk of death. Not all vital statistics agencies recognize therapeutic complication as a manner-of death classification and in that instance, the death should be classified as either natural or undetermined. The association of the death with medical therapy is indicated in descriptive terms by the certifier either in the "describe how injury occurred" section or Part I or Part II sections of the death certificate.

Accident as a manner-of-death classification may be applied in the case of the unexpected death from either the appropriate, inappropriate, or incorrect use or application of a device, procedure or medication. Diagnostic or screening procedures that cause perforation of non-diseased viscera or vasculature with subsequent sequela and death would be a general example warranting classification as accident. This same classification would apply in the case of administration of excessive or incorrect medication, improperly prepared medication, or failure to restart medication therapy in a hospitalized patient following surgery, as well. Use of *undetermined* manner-of-death classification may be necessary when it cannot be determined if a particular therapy was associated with the death, especially with a protracted hospital course in which other intervening medical interventions were performed. Rarely, homicidal manner-of-death classification would be applied in the case of a death resulting from the deliberate, gross and wanton action (manslaughter or murder) or inaction (medical neglect) by a medical caregiver or someone impersonating as a medical caregiver. Deaths due to euthanasia or assisted suicide may also be classified as homicide.

The following are 6 examples of peri-procedural or therapy-associated cause-of-death statements with brief scenarios included:

1. A 56 year-old man with a history of hypertension and coronary atherosclerosis with a remote myocardial infarct undergoes emergent, uncomplicated cholecystectomy for acute calculous and gangrenous cholecystitis. Shortly after the surgery, while recovering in the post-anesthesia care unit, he goes into cardiopulmonary arrest with resuscitation by protracted resuscitative efforts. He develops anoxic-ischemic encephalopathy followed by acute bronchopneumonia and respiratory failure for the remainder of the hospitalization, with a grim prognosis and little expectation for any functional recovery. After discussion with family, he is made do-not-resuscitate/comfort care only status and pronounced dead 24 hours after extubation. An autopsy reveals evidence of an uncomplicated cholecystectomy, lung consolidation, moderate left ventricular hypertrophy, moderate 3-vessel coronary atherosclerosis with acute intraplaque hemorrhage of one of the arteries, a 6.0 cm x 5.0 cm x 1.0 cm area of fibrosis of the left ventricle, and chronic hypertensive changes of the kidneys, all confirmed histologically. In light of the findings, the cause-of-death statement may be formulated as:

Part I. A. **Acute bronchopneumonia with respiratory failure**	Approximate interval: Onset to death **12 hours**
Due to (or as a consequence of): B. **Anoxic-ischemic encephalopathy following post-operative cardiopulmonary arrest with resuscitation**	**24 hours**
Due to (or as a consequence of): C. **Remote myocardial infarct**	**2 Years**
Due to (or as a consequence of): D. **Atherosclerotic coronary artery disease**	**10 years**
Part II. Other significant conditions contributing to death but not resulting in the underlying cause given in Part I **Emergent cholecystectomy for acute calculous and gangrenous cholecystitis**	
	Manner of Death **Natural**

This scenario describes a sudden death caused by chronic natural disease with known lethal potential and with acute coronary artery changes, in the setting of an intervening, uncomplicated surgery for a different natural disease condition. Coronary vasospasm with myocardial ischemia and arrhythmia are reasonable mechanisms of death that can be opined.

2. An 86 year-old woman with a 30-year history of hypertensive cardiovascular disease and a 15-year history of atrial fibrillation treated with warfarin develops a sudden severe headache and increasing confusion and unresponsiveness for 1 day prior to conveyance to the hospital. There is no history of a recent fall or other trauma. On hospital admission she is clinically hypertensive and imaging studies reveal massive intraparenchymal lobar hemorrhage with extension into the subarachnoid and ventricular spaces. An International Normalized Ratio test result is mildly supra-therapeutic. She is maintained on antihypertensive medications and her blood pressure remains stable in the high-normal range. She develops cerebral edema with herniation and dies 12 hours after admission. No autopsy is performed. The cause-of-death statement may be formulated as:

Part I.	Approximate interval: Onset to death
A. **Clinicopathologic sequelae of spontaneous acute intracerebral hemorrhage**	**36 hours**
Due to (or as a consequence of): B. **Therapeutic anticoagulation for atrial fibrillation**	**15 years**
Due to (or as a consequence of): C. **Hypertensive cardiovascular disease**	**30 years**
Due to (or as a consequence of): D.	
Part II. Other significant conditions contributing to death but not resulting in the underlying cause given in Part I	
	Manner of Death **Therapeutic complication (Natural)**

This scenario describes a known complication of anticoagulation medication therapy prescribed to prevent thromboembolic events caused by atrial fibrillation which is closely associated with hypertensive heart disease. Inclusion of all of the sequelae stemming from the hemorrhage (subarachnoid and intraventricular hemorrhage, cerebral edema with herniation) would exceed the permitted number of character spaces, hence usage of the all-encompassing terminology. Because cerebral hemorrhage may be traumatic in origin, it is important to differentiate clinically or by history whether or not the hemorrhage is traumatic or spontaneous as is specified in the example. Head trauma has different implications regarding manner-of-death determination and all trauma-associated deaths must be reported to the ME/C for investigation. Additionally, use of the word “intracerebral” is more anatomically specific and preferable rather than use of the word “intra-cranial” which is often used interchangeably in medical practice.

3. A 65 year-old woman with a history of schizophrenia stabilized with clozapine presents to the emergency department with a 3-day history of increasing abdominal distention and pain and difficulty with defecation. She additionally describes intermittent episodes of constipation with abdominal distention for the previous 6 months. She also has a history of longstanding hypertension and hyperlipidemia. Physical examination is notable for a distended abdomen with pain on palpation. While in the emergency room awaiting further clinical workup, she suddenly goes into cardiopulmonary arrest and could not be resuscitated with expiration 6 hours after arrival. The death is reported to the medical examiner who accepts jurisdiction but allows an autopsy to be performed at the hospital. Internal gross examination reveals markedly distended and dusky small and large intestines and copious semi-solid and firm fecal material is found within the stomach as well as the small and large intestines. Histologic examination of intestinal sections reveals acute hemorrhage, inflammation, and ischemic changes. Hypertensive and ischemic heart and kidney disease with moderate coronary atherosclerosis are additionally found and confirmed histologically. Blood samples drawn at the time of initial presentation are obtained and sent for toxicological testing with a resultant therapeutic level of clozapine:

Part I.	Approximate interval: Onset to death
A. **Toxic megacolon**	**3 days**
Due to (or as a consequence of): B. **Complications of clozapine medication therapy for schizophrenia**	**Years**
Due to (or as a consequence of): C.	
Due to (or as a consequence of): D.	
Part II.Other significant conditions contributing to death but not resulting in the underlying cause given in Part I **Hypertensive and atherosclerotic cardiovascular disease**	
	Manner of Death **Therapeutic Complication (Natural)**

This case is representative of a medication-related complication. Clozapine is known to confer gastric hypomotility and functional intestinal obstruction, most likely as a result from blockage of acetylcholine action on intestinal smooth muscle, an unintended side effect.

4. A 75 year-old woman with a history of Type II Diabetes Mellitus, hypertension, and end-stage renal disease (Stage IV) with weekly hemodialysis treatments is found at home unresponsive lying on her bedroom floor in a large pool of blood. A weak, rapid pulse, bradypnea, and a quarter-sized ulcerated defect with drainage of bloody fluid of the proximal left upper extremity are noted on initial assessment by paramedics and she is conveyed to the local hospital while resuscitation is continued. She becomes pulseless on arrival to the local hospital emergency department and despite continued resuscitative efforts, is pronounced dead shortly after arrival. A hospital autopsy is performed subsequent to consent of the legal next-of-in. At autopsy, a 7/8 x ½-inch cutaneous ulceration with full-thickness erosion of the subjacent subcutaneous arteriovenous dialysis graft along with drainage of bloody fluid are noted on the

proximal left upper extremity. Visceral pallor and hypertensive cardiovascular and renovascular disease are additionally found on internal gross examination. Inflammation, hemorrhage, and incomplete healing are seen in histological sections of the ulcer site. Diabetic nephropathy with changes of end-stage renal disease is confirmed histologically:

Part I. A. **Exsanguination**	Approximate interval: Onset to death **Minutes**
Due to (or as a consequence of): B. **Spontaneous acute rupture of arteriovenous graft of left upper extremity**	**Hours**
Due to (or as a consequence of): C. **End-stage renal disease (Stage IV) with therapeutic hemodialysis**	**Years**
Due to (or as a consequence of): D. **Type II Diabetes Mellitus with diabetic nephropathy**	**Years**
Part II. Other significant conditions contributing to death but not resulting in the underlying cause given in Part I **Hypertensive cardiovascular disease**	
	Manner of Death **Therapeutic Complication (Natural)**

This cause-of-death statement summarizes a known complication of long-term indwelling hemodialysis catheters in association with complicated diabetes mellitus and its associated effects on the healing process.

5. A 78 year-old woman with a history of stable hypertension develops barium peritonitis, *Escherichia coli* sepsis, and terminal multiple system organ failure over the period of a month's hospitalization, following perforation of her colon with massive spillage of barium following a diagnostic colonoscopy performed for moderate iron-deficiency anemia of uncertain etiology. Surgical intervention to repair the perforation is done after delayed discovery of the spillage heralded by a decline in her clinical status. No pathology or bleeding source is found in the examined colon during colonoscopy prior to the perforation. Autopsy and

histological examinations confirm the repaired colonic perforation, barium peritonitis and pathological changes of multi-organ failure in addition to mild hypertensive cardiovascular disease. The cause-of-death statement may appear as:

Part I.	Approximate interval: Onset to death
A. **Multiple system organ failure**	**7 days**
Due to (or as a consequence of): B. **Escherichia coli sepsis**	**3 weeks**
Due to (or as a consequence of): C. **Iatrogenic colonic perforation during diagnostic colonoscopy with barium peritonitis**	**4 weeks**
Due to (or as a consequence of): D.	
Part II. Other significant conditions contributing to death but not resulting in the underlying cause given in Part I **Iron-deficiency anemia of undetermined etiology** **Hypertensive cardiovascular disease**	
	Manner of Death **Accident**

This case is representative of the unanticipated outcome of a routine diagnostic colonoscopy in the setting of a compromised overall health status of stable chronic heart disease and anemia.

6. A 65 year-old man with a history of hypertension and hyperlipidemia has surgery to repair a symptomatic herniated L4-L5 vertebral disc. On post-operative days #2 and #3, the patient is treated with fluid resuscitation for tachycardia and mild anemia. At that time, his abdomen is noted to be distended but soft. On post-operative day #5, he is noted to be agitated and tachycardic. A surgical complication is suspected and he is taken back to the operating room for exploratory surgery. Retroperitoneal hemorrhage with massive intraperitoneal blood is encountered and a perforation of the abdominal aorta is found after removal of the blood. Repair of the aorta with multiple blood transfusions and fluid resuscitation are performed. Over the ensuing several hours, the patient develops signs of disseminated intravascular coagulation and multi-system organ

failure and goes into cardiac arrest with expiration despite resuscitative attempts. Due to the peri-procedural death circumstances, the death is reported and accepted under the jurisdiction of the local Medical Examiner's Office. Autopsy reveals cutaneous petechial hemorrhage, evidence of aortic repair, curetted lumbar disc at the same level as the aortic repair site, pale viscera, multivisceral petechial hemorrhage, changes of multi-organ failure, and hypertensive and atherosclerotic cardiovascular disease. A review of the post-operative progress notes and laboratory results reveals progressive decline in hemoglobin and hematocrit with reactive thrombocytosis, coinciding with elevation in heart rate:

Part I.	Approximate interval: Onset to death
A. **Disseminated intravascular coagulation with multi-system organ failure following emergent repair of aortic perforation**	**Hours**
Due to (or as a consequence of): B. **Exsanguination following iatrogenic perforation of aorta during lumbar discectomy**	**5 days**
Due to (or as a consequence of): C. **Herniation of lumbar disc with myelopathy**	**Years**
Due to (or as a consequence of): D.	
Part II. Other significant conditions contributing to death but not resulting in the underlying cause given in Part I **Hypertensive atherosclerotic cardiovascular disease**	
	Manner of Death **Accident**

This case represents an unanticipated fatal outcome in the setting of delayed recognition of the clinical signs of blood-loss anemia in the postoperative period.

8.6 Sample Natural Cause-of-Death Statements by Organ System

The following natural death scenarios are accompanied by suggested cause-of-death statements in deaths involving various organ systems. The manner of death in all cases is natural and thus the manner-of-death box has been intentionally omitted.

Neurological/Infectious Disease

A 45 year-old woman with a history of Acquired Immunodeficiency Syndrome caused by Human Immunodeficiency Virus (AIDS/HIV), non-compliant with her prescribed medication regimen, is found unresponsive at home. She was witnessed by family of having multiple seizure-like episodes followed by profound lethargy several days prior to death. Upon arrival and evaluation by paramedics, vital signs are absent and she is pronounced dead by the emergency medical control physician. At the local Medical Examiner's office, autopsy examination of the cachectic woman is additionally remarkable for cerebral congestion and ventricular hemorrhage associated with xanthochromic cerebral spinal fluid. Histological and immunohistochemical analysis of brain sections are performed which reveal evidence of HIV infection and Cytomegalovirus ventriculitis. Toxicology testing is later found to be non-contributory:

Part I.	Approximate interval: Onset to death
A. **Cytomegalovirus ventriculitis**	**Weeks**
Due to (or as a consequence of): B. **Profound immunodeficiency**	**Months**
Due to (or as a consequence of): C. **Acquired Immunodeficiency Syndrome**	**Decades**
Due to (or as a consequence of): D. **Human Immunodeficiency Virus infection**	**Decades**
Part II. Other significant conditions contributing to death but not resulting in the underlying cause given in Part I	

Neurological/Neurodegenerative

An 89 year-old woman has a diagnosis of Alzheimer's-type Dementia first diagnosed 10 years earlier. She also has a history of Type II Diabetes Mellitus and essential hypertension, both controlled with medications. Over the last 3-5 years she develops signs and symptoms of failure-to-thrive and an increase in her dementia symptoms. Due to her immobility, she additionally develops a Stage IV sacral decubital ulcer that becomes infected with Pseudomonas bacteria despite medical and surgical interventions and nursing home care. She has had episodic aspiration of food during monitored feedings and develops a fever, productive cough and decreased responsiveness. She dies of aspiration pneumonia with respiratory failure after a 3-day hospitalization. An autopsy is not performed:

<table>
<tr><td>Part I.

A. Aspiration pneumonia with respiratory failure</td><td>Approximate interval: Onset to death
Days</td></tr>
<tr><td>Due to (or as a consequence of):
B. Advanced Alzheimer's-type Dementia with failure-to-thrive</td><td>10 years</td></tr>
<tr><td>Due to (or as a consequence of):
C.</td><td></td></tr>
<tr><td>Due to (or as a consequence of):
D.</td><td></td></tr>
<tr><td colspan="2">Part II. Other significant conditions contributing to death but not resulting in the underlying cause given in Part I
Stage IV sacral decubital ulcer with Pseudomonas infection
Type II Diabetes Mellitus</td></tr>
</table>

Respiratory

A 33 year-old woman with a 10-year history of asthma well-controlled with her prescribed medication regimen and with only 2 admissions within the last 5 years for asthma exacerbation becomes unresponsive during a 911 call during which she reports sudden onset of wheezing and shortness of breath not relieved with her inhaler. There is no history of drug abuse and she had been recovering from a recent cold. Paramedics arrive to find her in respiratory arrest with a weakening pulse for which resuscitative efforts are unsuccessful. Upon verification of absence of vital signs, she is pronounced dead by the emergency medical control physician. Over-the-counter cold medications and her inhaler are found in close proximity to the decedent by an on-scene medicolegal death investigator who otherwise finds no illicit drugs, drug paraphernalia or signs of foul play. An autopsy is performed along with histological and toxicological testing at the local Coroner's Office. Cyanosis, hyperinflated lungs with mucous plugging, and acute and chronic asthmatic bronchial changes are found on histological examination, and there are no toxicological findings of significance:

Part I.	Approximate interval: Onset to death
A. **Acute bronchial asthma with acute respiratory failure**	**Minutes**
Due to (or as a consequence of): B. **Chronic asthmatic bronchitis**	**10 years**
Due to (or as a consequence of): C.	
Due to (or as a consequence of): D.	
Part II. Other significant conditions contributing to death but not resulting in the underlying cause given in Part I	

Cardiovascular

A 65 year-old man with a 25-year history of hypertension and hyperlipidemia, and a stable 2.0 cm abdominal aortic aneurysm diagnosed 10 years prior, presents to the emergency room with complaint of sudden, severe abdominal pain and distension for the past 6 hours. Physical examination is remarkable for tachycardia, hypotension, and a pulsatile distended abdomen. Subsequent ultrasonographic and confirmatory imaging studies reveal an aortic rupture. The patient goes into cardiac arrest while being prepped for an emergent laparoscopy and expires prior to surgery. At the family's request and consent, a hospital autopsy is performed. Massive liquid and clotted blood totaling 1050 ml are recovered from the abdominal cavity to unveil a 10.0 cm x 5.5 cm x 5.0 cm infrarenal abdominal aortic aneurysm. Severe, complicated atherosclerosis with mural thinning and fibrosis and an intimal tear with a subjacent 1.5 cm adventitial rupture site are additionally found. Findings of marked cardiomegaly with concentric left ventricular hypertrophy, mild to moderate coronary atherosclerosis, and granular renal cortices confirm the history of hypertension. The gross pathological findings are confirmed on examination of histological sections:

Part I. A. **Hemoperitoneum**	Approximate interval: Onset to death **6 Hours**
Due to (or as a consequence of): B. **Abdominal aortic aneurysm with spontaneous acute rupture**	**10 years**
Due to (or as a consequence of): C. **Atherosclerotic cardiovascular disease**	**25 years**
Due to (or as a consequence of): D.	
Part II. Other significant conditions contributing to death but not resulting in the underlying cause given in Part I **Hypertensive cardiovascular and renovascular disease**	

Gastrointestinal

A 55 year-old man with a history of chronic alcoholism and chronic back pain self-treated over the years with an over-the-counter non-steroidal anti-inflammatory medication (NSAID), had complaints of episodic abdominal pain, bloody sputum and bloody stool for several months duration. He is conveyed to the local hospital and admitted. He goes into cardiac arrest during the workup of the source of his bleeding and could not be resuscitated. A hospital autopsy is performed. External examination was notable for pallor of the conjunctiva and nailbeds and abdominal distention. Internal examination reveals 750 ml of intra-gastric blood and a full-thickness 3.5 cm in diameter duodenal ulcer with erosion of the underlying gastroduodenal artery. Fluid and clotted blood admixed with feces fill the entire length of the small and large intestines and visceral pallor is marked. The liver is mildly enlarged and fatty. Changes of moderate to severe spinal osteoarthritis are noted. Clinical toxicological testing reveals a therapeutic concentration of an NSAID and a 0.08 g/dL ethanol concentration. Moderate hypertensive and atherosclerotic cardiovascular disease is additionally found. Gross cardiovascular, hepatic, and gastric pathologies are all confirmed histologically:

Part I.	Approximate interval: Onset to death
A. **Acute upper gastrointestinal hemorrhage**	**Days**
Due to (or as a consequence of): B. **Peptic duodenal ulcer with erosion of gastroduodenal artery**	**Months**
Due to (or as a consequence of): C.	
Due to (or as a consequence of): D.	
Part II. Other significant conditions contributing to death but not resulting in the underlying cause given in Part I **Spinal osteoarthritis with analgesic medication therapy** **Chronic alcoholism with hepatic steatosis** **Hypertensive atherosclerotic cardiovascular disease**	

Endocrine

1. A 35 year-old woman with history of only a 2-day complaint of chest pain and shortness of breath is found obtunded at home. She is conveyed to the hospital and admitted to the cardiac intensive care unit and is diagnosed with an acute myocardial infarct. Eight hours into the admission and prior to a complete clinical workup to determine the cause of her infarct, she goes into cardiac arrest and despite resuscitative efforts is pronounced dead. Due to death occurring within 24 hours of admission in an otherwise young healthy woman, the death is reported and accepted by local Medical Examiner's Office. An autopsy confirms the acute myocardial infarct of the anterolateral left ventricle in addition to atherosclerotic stenosis with thrombosis of the left anterior descending coronary artery. Additionally, marked enlargement of the thyroid and thymus glands and marked atrophy of the adrenal glands are found. Microscopic examination of histological sections of thyroid and thymus glands reveal hyperplasia with lymphoplasmacytic infiltrates and corresponding cortical atrophy is found upon microscopic examination of adrenal gland sections. Serological testing on postmortem blood samples reveal markedly elevated thyroid hormone markers with evidence of hypothalamic negative feedback, and profound hypocortisolemia:

Part I.	Approximate interval: Onset to death
A. **Acute left ventricular myocardial infarct**	**2 days**
Due to (or as a consequence of): B. **Coronary arterial thrombosis of the left anterior descending coronary artery**	**Days**
Due to (or as a consequence of): C. **Atherosclerotic coronary artery disease**	**Years**
Due to (or as a consequence of): D.	
Part II. Other significant conditions contributing to death but not resulting in the underlying cause given in Part I **Probable Polyglandular Autoimmune Syndrome Type II**	

2. A 45 year-old woman with a history of hypertension, hyperlipidemia, longstanding Type I Diabetes Mellitus and non-compliance with her prescribed medication regimen is found obtunded at home. She was noted to have decreased responsiveness for the past 36 hours. 911 is called and emergency medical technicians arrive to find the woman with tachypnea, tachycardia, hypotension, and a fingerstick glucose reading of >500 mg/dL. Resuscitation efforts are initiated en route to the hospital. Clinical evaluation upon admission revealed a deteriorating clinical status with evidence of profound metabolic acidosis. She expires 6 hours after admission. The death is reported to the local medical examiner who declines jurisdiction. A hospital autopsy is not performed:

Part I.	Approximate interval: Onset to death
A. **Diabetic ketoacidosis**	**Hours**
Due to (or as a consequence of): B. **Insulin Dependent Diabetes Mellitus**	**Years**
Due to (or as a consequence of): C.	
Due to (or as a consequence of): D.	
Part II. Other significant conditions contributing to death but not resulting in the underlying cause given in Part I **Hypertension** **Hyperlipidemia**	

Genitourinary

A 25 year-old woman with a 2-week history of pelvic pain, fatigue, and increased girth is found dead at home. She has had 2 intervening hospital visits for the same complaint and after negative pregnancy testing was confirmed, she was sent home with narcotic analgesic medication. She is conveyed to the local Medical Examiner's office where an autopsy is performed. The autopsy reveals 1200 ml of old-appearing blood within the pelvic cavity, visceral pallor, and a pinpoint hemorrhagic defect of the right ovary. The endometrial cavity contains menstrual-type blood. A hemorrhagic corpus luteum cyst with acute and chronic inflammation and hemosiderin-laden macrophages is found on microscopic examination of the pathologic ovary. There is no histological evidence of early pregnancy on examination of ovarian and uterine sections:

Part I.	Approximate interval: Onset to death
A. **Hemoperitoneum**	**Days**
Due to (or as a consequence of): B. **Spontaneous acute rupture of right ovarian hemorrhagic corpus luteum cyst**	**2 weeks**
Due to (or as a consequence of): C.	
Due to (or as a consequence of): D.	
Part II. Other significant conditions contributing to death but not resulting in the underlying cause given in Part I	

Multisystem-Inflammatory

A 45 year-old man with a 2-year history of idiopathic arrhythmogenic cardiomyopathy treated with an implantable cardioverter defibrillator device (ICD) and medication presents to the emergency department with continuous shocks from his device. He goes into cardiac arrest shortly after arrival and cannot be resuscitated and is pronounced dead. A hospital autopsy is performed which includes an in-situ interrogation of the ICD device by the proprietary technician. Recordings of multiple continuous shock attempts for runs of ventricular fibrillation are found and the device is found to otherwise be functioning normally according to specifications. Gross examination of the heart reveals multiple, tan, soft, ill-defined, intramural biventricular lesions and absence of coronary artery disease. Multiple, tan, rubbery nodular lesions ranging from 0.3cm up to 0.8 cm in diameter are found throughout the lungs, liver, and spleen. Marked pulmonary hilar lymphadenopathy is additionally evident. Histological examination with histochemical staining of sections taken from lesional tissues reveals multivisceral sarcoidosis with extensive cardiac involvement:

Part I.	Approximate interval: Onset to death
A. **Ventricular fibrillation arrest with sudden cardiac death**	**Minutes**
Due to (or as a consequence of): B. **Cardiac sarcoidosis**	**Years**
Due to (or as a consequence of): C.	
Due to (or as a consequence of): D.	
Part II. Other significant conditions contributing to death but not resulting in the underlying cause given in Part I **Multivisceral sarcoidosis**	

<u>Multisystem-Malignancy</u>

A 65 year-old woman with a history of only hypertension experiences sudden onset of shortness of breath and called 911. Emergency medical technicians arrive to find her in respiratory distress and she is conveyed to the hospital. Diagnosis upon admission and initial clinical evaluation is that of respiratory failure with deteriorating vital signs terminating with cardiorespiratory arrest, within 1 hour after admission. The death is reported to the local Coroner who assumes jurisdiction over the death but allows an autopsy to be performed by the hospital autopsy pathologist. The autopsy reveals widely metastatic poorly-differentiated adenocarcinoma of unknown primary site, a saddle pulmonary arterial thromboembolus, and organizing thrombus of the bilateral popliteal veins:

Part I.	Approximate interval: Onset to death
A. **Pulmonary arterial thromboembolism**	**Hours**
Due to (or as a consequence of): B. **Deep vein thrombosis of bilateral lower extremities**	**Days**
Due to (or as a consequence of): C. **Metastatic adenocarcinoma, unknown primary site**	**Years**
Due to (or as a consequence of): D.	
Part II. Other significant conditions contributing to death but not resulting in the underlying cause given in Part I	

Autoimmune Inflammatory/Infectious disease

A 58 year-old man has a 10 year-history of Multiple Sclerosis over which time he develops quadriplegia and has been confined to a bed for the last year. His paralysis is further complicated by neurogenic bladder requiring indwelling urinary bladder catheterization and by Stage IV decubital ulcers with recent treatment for osteomyelitis caused by skin bacteria. He has had repeat *Escherichia coli* urinary tract infections over the last 5 years requiring hospitalization and antibiotic treatment. He also has a history of hypertensive cardiovascular disease, Peripheral Artery Disease, and Type II Diabetes Mellitus that has been stable on his prescribed medication regimen. More recently, he has had several days of increasing malaise and cloudy, dark urine noted in his drainage bag. He is hospitalized and diagnosed with *Escherichia coli* urosepsis and despite treatment develops signs of systemic inflammation and multi-system organ failure over the ensuing days. He is made DNR-CC status and expires shortly after removal from mechanical life supports. An autopsy is not performed:

Part I.	Approximate interval: Onset to death
A. **Clinicopathologic sequelae of Escherichia coli urosepsis**	Days
Due to (or as a consequence of): B. **Neurogenic bladder with chronic urinary tract infection**	**5-10 years**
Due to (or as a consequence of): C. **Multiple Sclerosis with quadriplegia**	**10 years**
Due to (or as a consequence of): D.	
Part II. Other significant conditions contributing to death but not resulting in the underlying cause given in Part I **Stage IV sacral decubiti with osteomyelitis. Type II Diabetes Mellitus. Hypertensive cardiovascular disease. Peripheral Artery Disease.**	

<u>Infectious</u>

An 8 year-old boy with a history of an upper respiratory infection 1 week prior has complaints of shortness of breath, tiredness, and chest pain for the past 2 days. He is found unresponsive but breathing and with a palpable pulse. Emergency medical services are summoned and the boy is found to be hypotensive and bradycardic. Resuscitation is initiated and he is conveyed to the hospital. Clinical evaluation upon admission reveals a diagnosis of acute congestive heart failure of uncertain etiology. Resuscitative therapies are continued but the boy goes into cardiac arrest before completion of a laboratory diagnostic workup. He is pronounced shortly thereafter. The death is reported to the local medical examiner who declines acceptance of jurisdiction as there are no reports or signs of foul play, trauma, or physical abuse. Consent for an autopsy is obtained from the parents. The autopsy reveals bilateral pleural effusions and a pale flabby heart with 4-chamber dilatation. Histological examination of multiple sections of heart reveal multifocal lymphohistiocytic infiltrates with myonecrosis. A nasopharyngeal swab later reveals adenovirus by culture and confirmed with polymerase chain reaction testing:

Part I.	Approximate interval: Onset to death
A. **Acute congestive heart failure**	**2 Days**
Due to (or as a consequence of): B. **Lymphocytic myocarditis**	**Days**
Due to (or as a consequence of): C. **Adenoviral upper respiratory infection**	**1 week**
Due to (or as a consequence of): D.	
Part II. Other significant conditions contributing to death but not resulting in the underlying cause given in Part I	

The above sample cause-of-death statements capture the essence of the disease conditions and processes leading to each patient's terminal decline and death. A medically understood, logical, cause-and-effect relationship exists between the lines in Part I and is not just a mere list of the patient's signs, symptoms or medical diagnoses. Part II includes medical conditions that either in-and-of themselves are not causally linked to items listed in Part I or are otherwise recognized risk factors. Inclusion of items in Part II provides a more complete picture of the patient's overall compromised health status. Moreover, sequential ordering of the components of the disease conditions from most recent to farthest back in time when read from top to bottom is done, using only specific medical terminology while avoiding use of shorthand and vague abbreviations. Table 8.1 summarizes the essentials of death certification.

Proficiency in death certification is enhanced first by understanding the necessary and important uses of the death certificate. Legal next-of-kin, physicians, attorneys, insurance companies, scientists, researchers, and the general public are just of few of the groups of individuals who have a vested interest in its components. Vital statistics and health department professionals continue in their efforts to educate certifiers about the death certification process in a variety of different venues including convenient on-line learning platforms. Proficiency is also enhanced by planned, periodic group tutorials and self-assessments by those individuals who certify the vast majority of deaths, namely physicians and other authorized clinical practitioners. Integration of these activities into the curriculum of residency training in the primary care specialties must also be done. Earlier introduction to the concepts of cause and manner of death along with death investigation should be provided to medical students by way of scheduled in-person or webinar lectures or by way of required clinical rotation at medical examiners' and coroners' offices. All information contained within this text provides the foundation towards that end. A two-part self-assessment module appears in Appendices H and I and is provided as a useful measuring tool of comprehension in additional to serving as a continuing medical educational (CME) activity.

Figure 8.1 Sample US Standard Death Certificate

U.S. STANDARD CERTIFICATE OF DEATH

LOCAL FILE NO. STATE FILE NO.

NAME OF DECEDENT ____ For use by physician or institution

To Be Completed/ Verified By: FUNERAL DIRECTOR:

1. DECEDENT'S LEGAL NAME (Include AKA's if any) (First, Middle, Last) | 2. SEX | 3. SOCIAL SECURITY NUMBER

4a. AGE-Last Birthday (Years) | 4b. UNDER 1 YEAR: Months, Days | 4c. UNDER 1 DAY: Hours, Minutes | 5. DATE OF BIRTH (Mo/Day/Yr) | 6. BIRTHPLACE (City and State or Foreign Country)

7a. RESIDENCE-STATE | 7b. COUNTY | 7c. CITY OR TOWN

7d. STREET AND NUMBER | 7e. APT. NO. | 7f. ZIP CODE | 7g. INSIDE CITY LIMITS? ☐ Yes ☐ No

8. EVER IN US ARMED FORCES? ☐ Yes ☐ No | 9. MARITAL STATUS AT TIME OF DEATH ☐ Married ☐ Married, but separated ☐ Widowed ☐ Divorced ☐ Never Married ☐ Unknown | 10. SURVIVING SPOUSE'S NAME (If wife, give name prior to first marriage)

11. FATHER'S NAME (First, Middle, Last) | 12. MOTHER'S NAME PRIOR TO FIRST MARRIAGE (First, Middle, Last)

13a. INFORMANT'S NAME | 13b. RELATIONSHIP TO DECEDENT | 13c. MAILING ADDRESS (Street and Number, City, State, Zip Code)

14. PLACE OF DEATH (Check only one: see instructions)

IF DEATH OCCURRED IN A HOSPITAL: ☐ Inpatient ☐ Emergency Room/Outpatient ☐ Dead on Arrival

IF DEATH OCCURRED SOMEWHERE OTHER THAN A HOSPITAL: ☐ Hospice facility ☐ Nursing home/Long term care facility ☐ Decedent's home ☐ Other (Specify):

15. FACILITY NAME (If not institution, give street & number) | 16. CITY OR TOWN, STATE, AND ZIP CODE | 17. COUNTY OF DEATH

18. METHOD OF DISPOSITION: ☐ Burial ☐ Cremation ☐ Donation ☐ Entombment ☐ Removal from State ☐ Other (Specify): ____ | 19. PLACE OF DISPOSITION (Name of cemetery, crematory, other place)

20. LOCATION-CITY, TOWN, AND STATE | 21. NAME AND COMPLETE ADDRESS OF FUNERAL FACILITY

22. SIGNATURE OF FUNERAL SERVICE LICENSEE OR OTHER AGENT | 23. LICENSE NUMBER (Of Licensee)

To Be Completed By: MEDICAL CERTIFIER

ITEMS 24-28 MUST BE COMPLETED BY PERSON WHO PRONOUNCES OR CERTIFIES DEATH | 24. DATE PRONOUNCED DEAD (Mo/Day/Yr) | 25. TIME PRONOUNCED DEAD

26. SIGNATURE OF PERSON PRONOUNCING DEATH (Only when applicable) | 27. LICENSE NUMBER | 28. DATE SIGNED (Mo/Day/Yr)

29. ACTUAL OR PRESUMED DATE OF DEATH (Mo/Day/Yr) (Spell Month) | 30. ACTUAL OR PRESUMED TIME OF DEATH | 31. WAS MEDICAL EXAMINER OR CORONER CONTACTED? ☐ Yes ☐ No

CAUSE OF DEATH (See instructions and examples)

32. PART I. Enter the chain of events--diseases, injuries, or complications--that directly caused the death. DO NOT enter terminal events such as cardiac arrest, respiratory arrest, or ventricular fibrillation without showing the etiology. DO NOT ABBREVIATE. Enter only one cause on a line. Add additional lines if necessary.

Approximate interval: Onset to death

IMMEDIATE CAUSE (Final disease or condition ——> resulting in death) a. ____
Due to (or as a consequence of):

Sequentially list conditions, if any, leading to the cause listed on line a. Enter the **UNDERLYING CAUSE** (disease or injury that initiated the events resulting in death) LAST

b. ____
Due to (or as a consequence of):

c. ____
Due to (or as a consequence of):

d. ____

PART II. Enter other significant conditions contributing to death but not resulting in the underlying cause given in PART I

33. WAS AN AUTOPSY PERFORMED? ☐ Yes ☐ No

34. WERE AUTOPSY FINDINGS AVAILABLE TO COMPLETE THE CAUSE OF DEATH? ☐ Yes ☐ No

35. DID TOBACCO USE CONTRIBUTE TO DEATH? ☐ Yes ☐ Probably ☐ No ☐ Unknown

36. IF FEMALE:
☐ Not pregnant within past year
☐ Pregnant at time of death
☐ Not pregnant, but pregnant within 42 days of death
☐ Not pregnant, but pregnant 43 days to 1 year before death
☐ Unknown if pregnant within the past year

37. MANNER OF DEATH
☐ Natural ☐ Homicide
☐ Accident ☐ Pending Investigation
☐ Suicide ☐ Could not be determined

38. DATE OF INJURY (Mo/Day/Yr) (Spell Month) | 39. TIME OF INJURY | 40. PLACE OF INJURY (e.g., Decedent's home; construction site; restaurant; wooded area) | 41. INJURY AT WORK? ☐ Yes ☐ No

42. LOCATION OF INJURY: State: City or Town:
Street & Number: Apartment No.: Zip Code:

43. DESCRIBE HOW INJURY OCCURRED:

44. IF TRANSPORTATION INJURY, SPECIFY:
☐ Driver/Operator
☐ Passenger
☐ Pedestrian
☐ Other (Specify)

45. CERTIFIER (Check only one):
☐ Certifying physician-To the best of my knowledge, death occurred due to the cause(s) and manner stated.
☐ Pronouncing & Certifying physician-To the best of my knowledge, death occurred at the time, date, and place, and due to the cause(s) and manner stated.
☐ Medical Examiner/Coroner-On the basis of examination, and/or investigation, in my opinion, death occurred at the time, date, and place, and due to the cause(s) and manner stated.

Signature of certifier: ____

46. NAME, ADDRESS, AND ZIP CODE OF PERSON COMPLETING CAUSE OF DEATH (Item 32)

47. TITLE OF CERTIFIER | 48. LICENSE NUMBER | 49. DATE CERTIFIED (Mo/Day/Yr) | 50. **FOR REGISTRAR ONLY**- DATE FILED (Mo/Day/Yr)

To Be Completed By: FUNERAL DIRECTOR

51. DECEDENT'S EDUCATION-Check the box that best describes the highest degree or level of school completed at the time of death.
☐ 8th grade or less
☐ 9th - 12th grade; no diploma
☐ High school graduate or GED completed
☐ Some college credit, but no degree
☐ Associate degree (e.g., AA, AS)
☐ Bachelor's degree (e.g., BA, AB, BS)
☐ Master's degree (e.g., MA, MS, MEng, MEd, MSW, MBA)
☐ Doctorate (e.g., PhD, EdD) or Professional degree (e.g., MD, DDS, DVM, LLB, JD)

52. DECEDENT OF HISPANIC ORIGIN? Check the box that best describes whether the decedent is Spanish/Hispanic/Latino. Check the "No" box if decedent is not Spanish/Hispanic/Latino.
☐ No, not Spanish/Hispanic/Latino
☐ Yes, Mexican, Mexican American, Chicano
☐ Yes, Puerto Rican
☐ Yes, Cuban
☐ Yes, other Spanish/Hispanic/Latino (Specify) ____

53. DECEDENT'S RACE (Check one or more races to indicate what the decedent considered himself or herself to be)
☐ White
☐ Black or African American
☐ American Indian or Alaska Native (Name of the enrolled or principal tribe) ____
☐ Asian Indian
☐ Chinese
☐ Filipino
☐ Japanese
☐ Korean
☐ Vietnamese
☐ Other Asian (Specify) ____
☐ Native Hawaiian
☐ Guamanian or Chamorro
☐ Samoan
☐ Other Pacific Islander (Specify) ____
☐ Other (Specify) ____

54. DECEDENT'S USUAL OCCUPATION (Indicate type of work done during most of working life. DO NOT USE RETIRED).

55. KIND OF BUSINESS/INDUSTRY

REV. 11/2003

Figure 8.2 Death Certificate from the State of Ohio

Reg. Dist. No. 18

Primary Reg. Dist. No. 1804

Registrar's No.

VITAL STATISTICS

CERTIFICATE OF DEATH

Type or print in permanent blue or black ink

State File No.

241327

DECEDENT

1. Decedent's Legal Name (Include AKA's if any) (First Middle, LAST, suffix)
2. Sex
3. Date of Death (Mo/Day/Year)
4. Social Security Number
5a. Age (Years)
5b. Under 1 Year: Months | Days
5c. Under 1 day: Hours | Minutes
6. Date of Birth (Mo/Day/Year)
7. Birthplace (City and State or Foreign Country)
8a. Residence State
8b. County
8c. City or Town
8d. Street and Number
8e. Apt. No.
8f. Zipcode
8g. Inside City Limits?
9. Ever in US Armed Forces?
10. Marital Status at Time of Death
11. Surviving Spouse's Name (If wife, give name prior to first marriage)
12. Decedent's Education
13. Decedent of Hispanic Origin
14. Decedent's Race
15. Father's Name
16. Mother's Name (prior to first marriage)
17a. Informant's Name
17b. Relationship to Decedent
17c. Mailing Address (Street and Number, City, State, Zip Code)
18a. Place of Death
18b. Facility Name (If not institution, give street & number)
18c. City or Town, State and Zip Code
18d. County of Death

DISPOSITION

19. Signature of Funeral Service Licensee or Other Agent
20. License Number (of licensee)
21. Name and Complete Address of Funeral Facility
22a. Method of Disposition
22b. Date of Disposition
22c. Place of Disposition (Name of Cemetery, Crematory, or other place)
22d. Location (City/Town and State)

REGISTRAR

23. Registrar's Signature
24. Date Filed
25a. Name of Person Issuing Burial Permit
25b. District No.
25c. Date Burial Permit Issued

CERTIFIER

26a. Certifier (Check only one)

☐ Certifying Physician
To the best of my knowledge, death occurred at the time, date, and place; and due to the cause(s) and manner stated.

☐ Coroner
On the basis of examination and/or investigation, in my opinion, death occurred at the time, date, and place; and due to the cause(s) and manner stated.

26b. Time of Death
26c. Date Pronounced Dead (Mo/Day/Year)
26d. Was case referred to coroner?
26e. Signature and Title of Certifier
26f. License number
26g. Date Signed
27. Name (Last, First, Middle) and Address of Person who Completed Cause of Death

CAUSE OF DEATH

28. Part I. Enter the disease, injuries, or complications that caused the death. Do not enter the mode of dying, such as cardiac or respiratory arrest, shock, or heart failure. List only one cause on each line. Type or print in permanent blue or black ink.

Approximate Interval Between Onset and Death

Immediate Cause (Final disease or condition resulting in death) a

Sequentially list conditions, if any, leading to immediate cause. b. Due to (or as Consequence of)

c. Due to (or as Consequence of)

Enter Underlying Cause (Disease or injury that initiated events resulting in a death) d. Due to (or as Consequence of)

Part II. Other significant conditions contributing to death but not resulting in the underlying cause given in Part I.

29a. Was An Autopsy Performed?
29b. Were Autopsy Findings Available Prior To Completion Of Cause of Death?
30. Did Tobacco Use Contribute to Death?
31. If Female, Pregnancy Status
32. Manner of Death
33a. Date of Injury (Mo/Day/Year)
33b. Time of Injury
33c. Place of Injury (e.g., Decedent's home, construction site, restaurant, wooded area)
33d. Injury at Work?
33e. Location of Injury (Street and Number or Rural Route Number, City or Town, State)
33f. Describe How Injury Occurred:
33g. If Transportation Injury, Specify:

HEA 2724 Rev. 01/07

Table 8.1 Essentials of Certification for Natural Deaths

Review death reporting laws in your State
Consult with the local ME/C for equivocal death circumstances
Review the requirements and the process of certification and registration
Review the structure and the terminology of the cause-of-death section
Enter the cause-of-death statement legibly on handwritten forms
Use etiologically specific medical terminology
Refrain from use of accusatory or derogatory terminology
Avoid common errors
Avoid use of terminology indicative of injury or intoxication
Verify that a sequential and logical order exists between 2 or more lines in Part I
Verify that statements logically correspond to the listed time intervals in Part I
Verify selection of "Natural" for the manner-of-death classification

References

1. Model State Vital Statistics Act and Model State Vital Statistics Regulations 2011 Revision. Available at: www.naphsis.org/Documents/FinalMODELLAWSeptember72011.pdf. Accessed 7/17/2016.

2. Moriyama IM, Loy RM, and Robb-Smitt AHT. Chapter 1: Evolution of Death Registration, In: History of the Statistical Classification of Diseases and Cause of Death. 2011. Available at: www.cdc.gov/nchs/data/misc/classification_diseases2011.pdf. Accessed 7/3/2016.

3. www.naphsis.org. Accessed 7/4/2016.

4. Nosologists: What Do They Do and Why Is It Important? Centers for Disease Control and Prevention. Available at: www.cdc.gov/nchs/features/nosologists.htm. Accessed 7/24/2016.

5. World Health Organization ICD Classifications. Available at: www.who.int/classifications/icd/en/. Accessed 1/20/2017.

6. Hoyert DI and Lima AR. Querying of death certificates in the United States. *Public Health Reports*. 2005; 120(3):288-93.

7. Instruction Manual Part 20, ICD-10 Cause of Death Querying, 1999. Available at: www.cdc.gov/nchs/data/dvs/20manual.pdf. Accessed: 11/19/2016.

8. Physicians' Handbook on Medical Certification of Death. Department of Health and Human Services, Centers for Disease Control and Prevention, National Center for Health Statistics. Available at: www.cdc.gov/nchs/data/misc/hb_cod.pdf. Accessed 7/24/2016.

9. Hanzlick R, editor. Cause of Death and the Death Certificate. 2006. College of American Pathologists (CAP).

10. Kircher T, Nelson J. Burdo H. The autopsy as a measure of accuracy of the death certificate. *N Engl J Med.* 1985;313(20):1263-69.

11. Nielsen GP, Bjornsson J, Jonasson JG. The accuracy of death certificates: Implications for health statistics. *Virchow Arch (A)* 1991;419(2):143-46.

12. Pritt BS, Hardin NJ, Ricmond JA, and Shapiro SL. Death certification errors at an academic institution. *Arch Pathol Lab Med.* 2005;129(11):1476-79.

13. Cambridge B and Cina SJ. The accuracy of death certificate completion in a suburban community. *Am J Forensic Med Pathol.* 2010;31(3):232-35.

14. Myers KA and Farquhar DRE. Improving the accuracy of death certification. *Canadian Medical Association.* 1998;158(10):1317-23.

15. National Notifiable Diseases Surveillance System (NNDSS). Available at: www.cdc.gov/nndss/. Accessed 10/9/2016.

16. Gill JR, Goldfeder LB, and Hirsch CS. Use of “therapeutic complication” as manner of death. *J Forensic Sci.* 2006;51(5):1127-33.

APPENDICES

Appendix A: Order of Legal Next-of-Kin

Defined as an individual's closest living blood relative, in order of precedence, to which benefits are dispersed, death notification is made, and transfer of the responsibility of handling the personal and legal matters of the decedent is done, *in the event that there is no spouse or partner.*

1. (Spouse or partner)
2. Adult children and their descendants
3. Parents
4. Adult grandchild
5. Adult siblings
6. Grandparent
7. Aunts, Uncles, Nieces, Nephews, Cousins, etc.
8. Guardian

Appendix B: Sample Report to the Medical Examiner/Coroner Form

Medical Record Number______________________ Date:__________

From:________________ Hospital Inpatient____ Emergency Room ____DOA____

Statement and Particulars in the Death of:________________________________

Home Address:__________________ Admission date_______ at_______ AM/PM

Conveyed to hospital by (ambulance, taxi, private car, etc.):_______ Unit #______

From:____(residence, public place, jail, etc.)

Address conveyed from:____

Race:___________ Occupation: _______________ Age____ Years____ Months____ Days:____

Married/Single/Widowed/Divorced:____
(circle one) (name and telephone # of surviving spouse or sig. other)

THE SECTION BELOW MUST BE COMPLETED IN FULL (DO NOT WRITE SEE CHART, LIST, ETC.)

Admitting Physician:_________________________________ MD/DO
Chief Complaint(s):____
Principal Diagnosis:____
Past Medical and Surgical History:____
Current Medical Disease:____
Prescription and/or Illicit Drugs used by patient:_______________________________________
Medications administered:____
Is death from NATURAL CAUSES? YES or NO
If no, manner injuries were received if known:_______________________________________
____
Therapy instituted (including any operative procedures):______________________________
____
Were any foreign bodies recovered? YES NO N/A
If the patient did not recover from anesthesia, was the patient conscious prior to induction?:
YES NO N/A
Death took place on the____ day of_____ month, 20___, at _______ AM/PM
In your opinion, what is the probable cause of death?:_________________________________
____
____
Pronouncing Physician:_____________________________ ________________________________
(printed name) (signature)

Appendix C: Sample Death Report and Release Form

Section I

Patient Name:_________________________________ Admit Date :____ Time:____ AM/PM

Expiration Date:_______ Time:______ AM/PM Pronouncing Physician:__________________

Unit location at expiration:___________________________

Next-of-kin/Family/Representative name:____

relationship:_________________________________

contact number:_________________________________

Section II

Medical Examiner/Coroner's (ME/C) case? Y/N

-If yes, has ME/C been called for removal? Y/N

Personal effects and valuables? Y/N (if yes, complete inventory/release form)

Autopsy requested? Y/N If yes, consent form completed? Y/N

-If ME/C case, has ME/C been notified of request? Y/N

Notifications:

Family/Representative	Y/N
Pastoral Care	Y/N
Attending Physician	Y/N
Consulting Physician(s)	Y/N
Security	Y/N
Organ/Tissue Procurement Organization	(required notification w/in 1 hour of death)

Section III

Body Release Authorization

Authorization to deliver to:____

(Funeral Home or Medical Examiner/Coroner)

The body of:____

(Patient)

Witness:___________________________ Signed:___________________________________

(Unit/Hospital Representative) (Family Member/Representative)

Date:__________________

Section IV

Body Release Verification

My signature below certifies that I have removed the deceased body from _________________

(medical facility)

X____________________________________ ____

(signature of Funeral Home, ME/C Representative) (name of Funeral Home, ME/C's Office)

X____________________________________ Date:_____________

(Witness Signature)

Appendix D: Death Reporting/Certification Flow Charts

Reportable Death → Report to ME/C → ME/C accepts jurisdiction

- inventory/secure personal effects and evidence (see Appendix E)
- leave medical devices in place
- notify family/representative
- complete death-related forms (see Appendices B and C)
- prepare body for transport

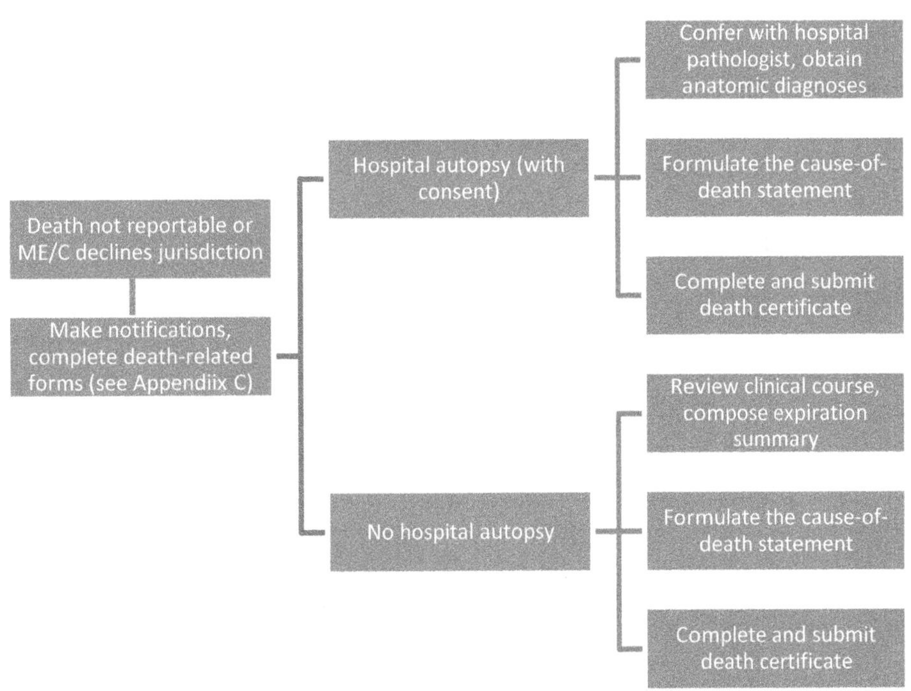

Appendix E: Sample Chain of Custody Form

Patient's Name and Medical Record Number______________________________

Number of Evidence Parcels Secured__________________________________

Clothing Bag ________________	Clothing Bag ____________________
Clothing Bag ________________	Clothing Bag____________________
Clothing Bag ________________	Clothing Bag ____________________
Clothing Bag ________________	Clothing Bag ____________________
Clothing Bag ________________	Clothing Bag ____________________
Miscellaneous item______________	Other____________________
Miscellaneous item _____________	Other ____________________

Evidence secured by:

________________________	____________________________
(Nurse/Physician/Security Officer-print name)	(Hospital/Facility and City)
________________________	________________
(Nurse/Physician/Security Officer Signature)	(Date and Time)

Evidence released by:

________________________	____________________________
(Nurse/Physician/Security Officer-print name)	(Hospital/Facility and City)
________________________	____________________________
(Nurse/Physician/Security Officer Signature)	(Date and Time)

Evidence released to:

________________________	____________________________
(ME/C Representative-print name)	(Agency)
________________________	________________
(ME/C signature)	(Date and Time)
________________________	____________________________
(Law Enforcement-print name/badge #)	(Agency)
________________________	________________
(Law Enforcement-signature)	(Date and Time)

Appendix F: Sample Autopsy Consent and Authorization Form (adapted from the College of American Pathologists' sample form)

Service:___________________
Attending Physician:___________________________
Date of death:____________ Time of death: __________AM/PM

I, (print name)_____________________, the (relationship to the deceased______________, being entitled by law to control the disposition of the remains, hereby request the pathologist of (name of Hospital)______________________________ to perform an autopsy on the body of said deceased. I understand that any diagnostic information gained from the autopsy will become part of the decedent's medical record and will be subject to applicable laws.

Retention of Organs/Tissues:

I authorize the removal, examination, and retention of organs, tissues, prosthetic and implantable devices, and fluids as the pathologist deems proper for diagnostic, educational, quality improvement and research purposes. I further agree to the eventual disposition of these materials as the pathologist or the hospital determines or as required by law. This consent does not extend to the removal or use of any of these materials for the transplantation or similar purposes. I understand that organs and tissues not needed for diagnostic, educational, quality improvement, or research purposes will be sent to the funeral home or disposed of appropriately.

I understand that I may place limitations on both the extent of the autopsy and on the retention of organs, tissues, and devices. I understand that any limitations may compromise the diagnostic value of the autopsy and may limit the usefulness of the autopsy for educational, quality improvement, or research purposes. I have been given the opportunity to ask any questions that I may have regarding the scope or purpose of the autopsy.

Limitations:

__ None. Permission is granted for a complete autopsy with removal, examination and retention of materials as the pathologist deems proper for the purposes set forth above and for disposition of such material as the pathologist or hospital determine.

__ Permission is granted for an autopsy with the following limitations and conditions (specify):

____

____

________________________________	__________	__________AM/PM
Signature of person authorizing autopsy	Date	Time

__ Permission obtained by telephone

________________________________	________________________________
Signature of person obtaining permission	Printed name of person obtaining permission
________________________________	________________________________
Signature of witness	Printed name of witness

Appendix G: Sample Hospital Autopsy Report

Case Scenario: A 30 year-old obese Caucasian woman develops respiratory distress and chest pain while watching television at home. One week prior, she had complaints of intermittent wheezing and productive cough in addition to right calf tightness which prompted a trip to the emergency room where she was evaluated, received breathing treatments and was discharged to home. She had no past medical history but had begun taking prescribed oral birth control pills 2 months prior. She is conveyed to the hospital and upon arrival develops worsening respiratory symptoms and clinical signs of hypoxia requiring intubation. She goes into cardiac arrest and despite resuscitative efforts expires while in the emergency department prior to a complete clinical diagnostic workup. The death is reported to the Medical Examiner who accepts jurisdiction but allows an autopsy to be performed at the hospital.

Metropolitan Hospitals

Department of Pathology
678 Market Street, Anytown, Anystate 65412
Phone: 123-456-7890 www.MetropolitanHospitals.org

Patient Name: Anna Smith
Medical Record #: 23456789 **Encounter #:** 7654321
DOB: 10/01/1986 (Age: 30 years)
Sex: Female **Race:** Caucasian
Date of Service: 11/01/2016
Location: Emergency Department

Postmortem Record

Date and time of death: 11/01/2016, 12:00 PM **Autopsy #:** 16-35AN
Autopsy date and time: 11/2/2016, 12:00 PM **Prosector:** James Jones DO, PGY-3
Hours Postmortem: 24 **Senior Pathologist:** Helen Johnson MD
Restrictions: None
Identification Method: Hospital ID band comparison to medical records
Observers: None

FINAL CLINICAL AND ANATOMIC DIAGNOSIS

I. Deep venous thrombosis of right lower extremity, organizing
- A. Pulmonary arterial thromboembolism, acute
  1. Pulmonary congestion and edema, moderate
  2. Right ventricular dilatation, severe
- B. Hypoxia with respiratory failure (clinical)

II. Obesity (Body Mass Index 33)

III. Hepatomegaly (2100 grams) with steatohepatitis

IV. Uterine leiomyomata

V. Therapeutic interventions:
- A. Endotracheal intubation
- B. Venipunctures with intravascular catheter placements
- C. Electrocardiogram and defibrillation pad placements
- D. Indwelling urinary bladder catheter placement
- E. Resuscitative chest compression(s) with cutaneous and skeletal injuries

Cause-of-Death Statement:

Pulmonary arterial thromboembolism
Due to: Deep venous thrombosis of right lower extremity

Other Significant Conditions: Obesity. Non-alcoholic steatohepatitis. Oral contraceptive use.

Clinical Diagnosis/History:

This was a 30 year-old female with recent initiation of oral contraception medication and no significant past medical history who presented with symptoms of respiratory compromise and found clinically to have signs of hypoxia. Of note was a recent hospital visit for similar symptomatology in addition to non-specific but relevant symptoms of the right lower extremity. Her respiratory status worsened requiring intubation. Sudden cardiac arrest soon followed with expiration despite resuscitative efforts prior to complete clinical diagnostic workup.

Clinicopathologic Summary and Comment:

Based on the autopsy findings, the cause of death is as a result of pulmonary arterial thromboembolism of recent formation caused by deep venous thrombosis, in the context of recent initiation of oral contraception in an obese woman and interim symptoms indicative of but not specific for an evolving acute medical condition. It is opined further that the recent use of oral contraceptive medication in combination with obesity and non-alcoholic steatohepatitis constitute risk factors associated with the development of a hypercoagulable state which separately or in combination conferred the development of deep venous thrombosis heralded by an increase in calf circumference. The patient reported right calf tightness which was consistent with the autopsy findings. The finding of pulmonary congestion and edema represent physiologic derangements and the anatomic correlate to the clinically evident hypoxia. The terminal mechanism of death was likely right-sided heart failure as revealed by right ventricular dilatation caused by thrombotic obstruction of the pulmonary arterial circulation.

Additional Studies Performed:

Histology:
Routine histology tissue blocks and sections of thromboembolic clot are submitted. See microscopic description.

AUTOPSY PROTOCOL

EXTERNAL EXAMINATION:

The body is that of a well-developed, obese Caucasian female whose appearance is compatible with the state age of 30 years. The body weighs 198 pounds and is 65 inches in length. The body is cool to palpation. The body is in full rigor mortis with posterior slightly blanching livor mortis.

The scalp hair is brown and up to 12 inches in length. The eyes are brown. The corneas are unremarkable. The sclerae are congested. Multiple piercings are of each ear lobe. The nose and lips are unremarkable. The teeth are natural and in good condition. The neck is unremarkable. The chest and breasts are symmetrical and the breasts are without palpable masses. The abdomen is markedly protuberant with a Grade 2 panniculus. The external genitalia are well-developed and symmetrical. A hospital identification bracelet with the decedent's name is around the left wrist. Red and white nail polish is upon the fingernails and toenails. The calves are asymmetrical in circumference: Right 17 ½ inches, Left 15 inches.

IDENTIFYING MARKS AND SCARS:

1. A multicolored tattoo of a rose is of the left shoulder.
2. A 1 ½ inch irregular scar is of the right knee.

EXTERNAL AND INTERNAL EVIDENCE OF RECENT THERAPY:

1. An oral endotracheal tube in inserted into the trachea superior to the carina.
2. An intravascular catheter is of the right antecubital fossa and of the left wrist.
3. Multiple venipunctures are of the left antecubital fossa and dorsal left hand.
3. Twelve electrocardiogram pads are of the torso.
4. Defibrillation pads are present with associated underlying thermo-abrasive injury.

EXTERNAL AND INTERNAL EVIDENCE OF RECENT INJURY:

1. Of the mid chest is a cluster of multiple, curvilinear, red-brown **abrasion**s that overlie a 4 x 3 ½ inch area. Further internal examination reveals subcutaneous hemorrhage and sternal fracture with hemorrhage, at the 3rd rib level.
2. A ¾ X ½ inch purple-contusion is of the anterior and proximal thigh.

The injuries above, once having been stated, will not be repeated below.

INTERNAL EXAMINATION:

BODY CAVITIES: The body is opened by means of the usual Y-incision with subsequent removal of the chest plate. Evisceration is continued using the Ghon/en bloc method for removal of chest, abdominal, and pelvic organs. The thoracic and abdominal organs are in their normal anatomic positions. The body cavities contain no adhesions or abnormal collections of fluid. The thickness of the abdominal wall fat is a maximum of 2 ½ inches.

Organ weights:

Heart- 330 grams
Right lung- 560 grams
Left lung- 430 grams
Spleen- 325 grams
Liver- 2100 grams
Right kidney- 150 grams
Left kidney- 150 grams
Brain-1250 grams

NECK: The organs of the neck are examined in situ and the thyroid gland is resected separately. The soft tissues of the prevertebral fascia of the neck are unremarkable. The hyoid bone and larynx are intact.

CARDIOVASCULAR SYSTEM: The aorta and its major branches and the great vein are normally distributed. The intimal surface of the aorta is remarkable for frequent fatty streaks. The pericardium and epicardium are smooth, glistening, and unremarkable. The coronary arterial system is right dominant. The coronary ostia are patent. There is no grossly appreciable coronary atherosclerosis seen on multiple cross sections. There are no thrombi in the atrial or ventricles. The foramen ovale is probe patent. The atrial and ventricular septa are intact. The endocardium is smooth and unremarkable. The annular circumferences of the tricuspid, pulmonic, mitral, and aortic valves are 15.0 cm, 6.5 cm, 9.0 cm and 6.0 cm, respectively. The myocardium is red-brown and of normal consistency. Myocardial wall thicknesses: left ventricle-1.4 cm, septum-1.4 cm, and right ventricle-0.3 cm.

Longitudinal incision with dissection of the posterior bilateral lower extremities reveals red-tan, adherent, rubbery partially occlusive intravascular thrombus of the right popliteal vein.

RESPIRATORY SYSTEM: The upper airway is unobstructed. The laryngeal and tracheal mucosa is smooth and congested. The pleural surfaces are smooth and shiny. A cylindrical, red-tan, loosely adherent, occlusive saddle embolus is present with extension into the right and left pulmonary arteries. Dissection of the more distal segmental branches reveals no clot and the absence of intimal webs. The pulmonary veins are unremarkable. The major bronchi are unremarkable. The pulmonary parenchyma is dark-red and spongy. There is moderate vascular congestion and moderate pulmonary edema within all lobes of both lungs.

HEPATOBILIARY SYSTEM: The liver is enlarged with a smooth and glistening capsule. The parenchyma is dark-yellow and its consistency is soft and greasy. There is moderate congestion. The gall bladder contains 15 ml of green and slightly viscous fluid. There are no calculi. The extrahepatic biliary ducts are unremarkable, externally and internally.

DIGESTIVE SYSTEM: The esophageal mucosa is gray, wrinkled and unremarkable. The stomach contains 100 ml of a tan fluid admixed with multiple, irregular, brown meat fragments and green vegetable fragments. There are no tablets and capsules. The gastric mucosa has normal rugal folds and there are no ulcers. The small and large intestines are unremarkable and the large intestine contains soft, brown fecal material. The appendix is present. The pancreas is unremarkable externally and upon sectioning.

RETICULOENDOTHELIAL SYSTEM: The spleen is enlarged and congested with a thin, smooth, and intact capsule. The parenchyma is dark-red and soft. The lymph nodes are unremarkable. The thymus gland is not grossly apparent.

GENITOURINARY SYSTEM: The subcapsular surfaces of the kidneys are smooth. The cortices are of normal thickness. The calyces, pelves, and ureters are unremarkable. The urinary bladder is devoid of urine. The mucosal is gray, smooth and unremarkable. The urinary bladder wall is unremarkable.

The uterus is enlarged and sectioning reveals multiple subserosal and myometrial leiomyomatous nodules ranging from 1.0 cm up to 4.5 cm in diameter. All nodules have a homogenously tan appearance and rubbery consistency. A hemorrhagic corpus luteum is of the left ovary. The endometrium is thick, red-tan and velvety. The cervix and fallopian tubes are unremarkable externally and upon sectioning.

ENDOCRINE SYSTEM: The thyroid and adrenal glands are unremarkable externally and upon sectioning. The pituitary gland is unremarkable.

MUSCULOSKELETAL SYSTEM: The clavicles, ribs, pelvis, and vertebral column are unremarkable and without fractures. The diaphragm is intact.

BRAIN: The scalp, subgalea, and skull are unremarkable. The dura and dural sinuses are unremarkable. There are no epidural, subdural, or subarachnoid hemorrhages. The leptomeninges are thin and delicate. The cerebral hemispheres are symmetrical with an unremarkable gyral pattern and there is cortical vascular congestion. There is no evidence of herniation. The intracranial blood vessels have no grossly appreciable atherosclerosis. The cranial nerves are unremarkable. Sections throughout the cerebral hemispheres, brainstem, and cerebellum are unremarkable. There are no hemorrhages in the deep white matter or basal ganglia. The cerebral ventricles contain non blood.

SPINAL CORD: The spinal cord is not removed or examined.

Microscopic Description/Diagnosis:

HEART:	No pathological diagnosis, section of right and left ventricles
VASCULAR:	Antemortem intravenous thrombus with lines of Zahn hemosiderophages, and fibroblastic infiltration and recanalization at periphery, section of right popliteal vein with thrombus
LUNGS:	Antemortem, intra-arterial thromboembolic blood clot, with lines of Zahn, intimal proliferation, and focal early fibroblastic infiltration, section of arterial blood clot Acute congestion Hemorrhagic edema Numerous intra-alveolar debris-laden macrophages
LIVER:	Diffuse, panlobular macrovesicular steatosis, multifocal hepatocellular necrosis with acute and chronic reactive inflammation, and early portal bridging fibrosis
KIDNEYS:	Acute congestion Tubular autolysis
GENITOURINARY:	Leiomyoma, cellular variant
BRAIN:	No pathological diagnosis, section of cerebellum, hippocampus, and neocortex

Appendix H
Part I: Self-Assessment: General
(answers appear at the end of this exercise)

1. Which governmental entity requires by law the investigation of sudden, unexpected and unexplained deaths by the Medical Examiner or Coroner?

   A. Federal
   B. State
   C. City
   D. State Bar Association

2. All reportable deaths occurring within a medical facility are exempt from the Health Insurance Portability and Accountability Act-Privacy Rule. True or False?

3. A 35-year-old quadriplegic, who sustained spinal cord injury subsequent to a gunshot wound of the neck 15 years prior, has since been on mechanical ventilation. He dies of bronchopneumonia. His death does not have to be reported to the Coroner/Medical Examiner. True or False?

4. Which of the following death(s) is/are reportable to the Medical Examiner or Coroner? (circle all that apply)

   A. Patient with severe coronary artery disease recovering from a myocardial infarct with sudden death on hospital day #3
   B. Woman with Bipolar Disorder expires after 1 week of hospitalization for an acetaminophen overdose
   C. 45-year-old woman hospitalized 1 week for an asthma exacerbation due to bronchopneumonia with subsequent respiratory failure and death
   D. Elderly woman with congestive heart failure and chronic renal failure due to hypertensive heart disease, found expired in bed at the nursing home where she is recovering from a hip fracture
   E. 58 year-old man with diabetic nephropathy and end-stage kidney disease found unresponsive in his jail cell and pronounced dead 30 hours after hospitalization despite resuscitative efforts

5. A physician makes a yearly house call to her elderly patient for which she has provided care for the past 30 years. She is let in by the live-in caretaker. To her surprise, the patient, who usually greets her at the door, is in bed and is obtunded, emaciated, and appears dehydrated. During the physical examination, signs of dehydration and a Stage 3 sacral ulcer are additionally noted. The patient suddenly becomes unresponsive with a weak, thready pulse. The physician attempts CPR inclusive of use of her portable defibrillator but after several tries, the patient's vital signs become absent. She pronounces the patient dead. The live-in caretaker had abruptly left near the beginning of the examination. A neighbor arrives and tells the physician that she recently saw the caretaker and several acquaintances haul furniture and clothing out of the back door one night. The physician's professional responsibility is to:

A. Call the local funeral home to come get the patient and when the Funeral Director sends the death certificate for completion, certify the cause of death as "Probable dehydration due to failure-to-thrive" and the manner of death as "Natural"
B. Call the local funeral home to come get the patient. Hold off on signing the death certificate and hire a private detective to investigate the caretaker
C. Call the police and/or call and report the death to Coroner or Medical examiner

6. A 55 year-old woman recently had been complaining of chest pains to her co-worker. She has a known history of hyperlipidemia and has had 2 coronary artery stent placements. She is found slumped over at her desk in her office where she works as a supervisor for a chemical engineering and manufacturing company. Her cardiologist's card with contact information is found on her desk next to her. 911 is called and police and EMS respond. She is apneic and has a weak pulse and resuscitative efforts are initiated and continued en route to the hospital. Despite these efforts, she does not regain vital signs and is pronounced dead shortly after arrival. There are no signs of trauma. This death is reportable for what 2 reasons?

7. A 35-year-old female with pituitary insufficiency, status post remote surgical resection for Sheehan's syndrome, undergoes an elective splenectomy for splenomegaly which is completed without complication. She recovers in the Post-Anesthesia Care Unit (PACU) and in conveyed to the surgical floor. Several hours

later, on a routine nurse's check, she is discovered obtunded with a rapid heart rate and subsequently goes into cardiopulmonary arrest. A stat blood chemistry test reveals a sodium concentration of 185 mmol/L. The nurse realizes that the order to resume the patient's DDAVP medication after surgery had not been entered on the patient's chart by the physician. Despite resuscitative attempts, the patient expires. This death is reportable for what 2 reasons?

8. A 47-year-old on-duty physician collapses in the medical ward after sprinting up 6 flights of stairs in response to a page for a "code blue". He is found to be in cardiac arrest and cannot be resuscitated and is pronounced dead. This death needs reporting to the Coroner/Medical Examiner. True or False?

9. A middle-aged woman is conveyed by paramedics from home to the ER due to unresponsiveness. The emergency medical technician had performed a finger stick test which revealed a glucose level > 500 mg/dL. Her husband tells the emergency medical technician that she has diabetes and frequently skips insulin doses. Resuscitation is started and continued en route to the hospital. In the past year, she has had 2 admissions to the same hospital for complications of hyperglycemia. Despite resuscitation efforts, she is pronounced dead shortly after arrival in the ER. The attending ER physician is certain that she has died of diabetic ketoacidosis and is willing to sign the death certificate. This death is reportable to the Coroner/Medical Examiner. True or False?

10. All decedents that come under the jurisdiction of the Medical Examiner or Coroner will receive an autopsy. True or False?

11. Physicians in clinical practice are responsible for certifying which manner of death?

A. Accidental
B. Natural
C. Homicide
D. Suicide
E. All of the above

12. Collectively, clinical physicians and other authorized clinical practitioners complete fewer death certificates than forensic pathologists. True or False?

13. Certification of a patient's natural, non-reportable death by the clinician of record is optional. True or False?

14. Name the 2 general phases necessary to complete a death certificate.

15. The demographic and personal information sections on the death certificate are completed by the Funeral Director. True or False?

16. The cause-of-death statement is one of absolute medical certainty (>90%) that the disease and/or disease complication is what led to the death. True or False?

17. Once completed, the death certificate is final and the cause-of-death statement may not be amended at a future date. True or False?

18. The etiologically specific disease or disease condition that gives rise to one or more physiologic derangement(s) or non-specific process(es), terminating in death defines what?

19. Mechanisms of death are inherently etiologically specific. True or False?

20. On Part II of the Cause-of-Death section of the death certificate, other significant conditions refer to conditions that arose after or are a result of the underlying cause of death. True or False?

21. The 4 lines on Part I of the Cause-of-Death section of the death certificate are for listing up to 4 of the patient's most recently diagnosed medical conditions. True or False?

22. The inclusion of signs and symptoms is not permitted on the death certificate. True or False?

23. A patient with prolonged hospitalization for well-documented, natural, non-trauma-related chronic disease dies in the hospital after unsuccessful cardiopulmonary resuscitation performed by the cross-covering attending physician. The patient's regular attending physician is out of the country and will not return for 1 month. The next step for the cross-covering attending physician is to:

A. Wait for the patient's regular physician to return and have her certify the cause of death and sign the death certificate
B. Promptly certify the cause of death as accurately as possible and sign the death certificate
C. Don't certify the death or sign the death certificate; leave that to the Funeral Director
D. Don't certify the death or sign the death certificate; this death is reportable to the local Coroner or Medical Examiner

24. A 65-year-old man with a 2-day history of chest pain and chest pressure presents to the ER. He has a medical history of coronary artery disease. There is no interval or past history of trauma or drug use. An EKG shows ST segment elevation and ventricular tachycardia. Before blood can be drawn for cardiac enzymes, the man suddenly becomes unresponsive and goes into cardiac arrest. He could not be resuscitated after 25 minutes of resuscitative efforts and is pronounced dead. He is reported to the Coroner but the ER physician is willing to sign the death certificate and thus jurisdiction is not assumed by the Coroner. The death is designated as a "Report and Release" death by the Coroner. A reasonable cause-of-death statement in this case is:

A. "Probable" or "presumed acute myocardial infarct due to atherosclerotic coronary artery disease"
B. "Spontaneous rupture of cerebral artery aneurysm"
C. "Aortic dissection"
D. The death certificate cannot be completed without performance of an autopsy. The physician should contact the family to request that they consent to a hospital autopsy.

25. A 45-year-old with a history of long-standing hypertension dies in the CICU, 36 hours after admission. A hospital autopsy reveals left ventricular hypertrophy,

atherosclerosis and thrombosis with occlusion of the left anterior descending coronary artery, and an acute myocardial infarct of the anterolateral left ventricle. The other significant condition in this case is:

A. Atherosclerotic coronary artery disease
B. Essential hypertension
C. Acute myocardial infarct
D. Coronary artery thrombosis
E. None of the above

26. A 45-year-old woman with a history of hypertension and Insulin Dependent Diabetes Mellitus has been out of work for 6 months and no longer has medical insurance coverage. For the past 2 months, she has been unable to fill her insulin prescriptions and has been "stretching out" the doses of her last 2 bottles. She is found unresponsive in bed. 911 is called and EMS and police respond. EMS technicians find a weak pulse and slow, deep respirations. Resuscitation is initiated and continued en route to the hospital and in the ED. Initial blood tests are diagnostic for diabetic ketoacidosis. Despite resuscitative efforts the patient expires 26 hours after admission. A hospital autopsy with microscopic examination reveals mild to moderate hypertensive cardiovascular disease and diabetic nephropathy. What is the other significant condition in this case?

A. Insulin Dependent Diabetes Mellitus
B. Diabetic Ketoacidosis
C. Hypertensive cardiovascular disease
D. Peripheral neuropathy

27. A 55-year-old man has smoked 3 packs of cigarettes per day for the last 30 years. He recently had been diagnosed with severe emphysema and has been using home oxygen by nasal cannula. He had recent complaints of fever with cough productive of yellow sputum. He is found in respiratory distress at home. He is conveyed and admitted to the hospital with a diagnosis of respiratory failure and dies 3 days later. The legal next-of-kin requests a full autopsy. A hospital autopsy reveals heavy consolidated lungs (right lung 1000 grams, left lung 850 grams) and mild hypertensive heart disease. Microscopic examination is

significant for acute bronchopneumonia and severe pulmonary emphysema. What is the underlying cause of death?

A. Respiratory failure
B. Acute bronchopneumonia
C. Severe pulmonary emphysema
D. Hypertensive heart disease

28. A 55-year-old female with a history of uncontrolled hypertension is found collapsed at the bottom of the stairs at home. EMS respond to the unresponsive woman who is breathing but has markedly elevated blood pressure and heart rate. She is conveyed to the local hospital and upon admission her blood pressure is 200/100 and heart rate 120 bpm. She has a contusion with soft tissue swelling on her forehead. CT scanning reveals periventricular and intraventricular hemorrhage. Imaging studies of the head and neck reveal mild osteoarthritis of the cervical spine but no skull or cervical spine fracture. Despite resuscitative and supportive efforts, she expires 6 hours after admission. The death is reported to the Coroner who accepts jurisdiction but allows an autopsy to be performed at the admitting hospital subsequent to the family's request. Internal examination at autopsy reveals hemorrhagic necrosis of the right putamen and globus pallidus with extension to the periventricular white matter and associated hemorrhage into the lateral, 3rd and 4th ventricles. Findings consistent with hypertensive cardio- and renovascular disease are also noted. Microscopic examination later confirms all gross findings. The toxicology screening test is later found to be negative for drugs of abuse. What is the manner of death?

A. Natural
B. Accident
C. Homicide
D. Suicide

Part I: Self-Assessment/General- Answers and Reference/Explanation

1. B	Ch. 3(3.1)
2. True	Ch. 3(3.1)
3. False	Table 3.1
4. B, D, and E	Table 3.1, Ch. 7
5. C	Table 3.1
6. Sudden, work-related	Table 3.1
7. Sudden, Therapy-associated	Table 3.1
8. True	Table 3.1, work-related
9. True	Table 3.1, DAA
10. False	Ch. 6(6.4)
11. B	Ch. 8(Introduction)
12. False	Ch. 8(Introduction)
13. False	Ch. 8(Introduction)
14. Certification and Registration	Ch. 8(8.1)
15. True	Ch. 8(8.1)
16. False	Ch. 8(8.3)
17. False	Ch. 8(8.1)
18. Underlying cause of death	Ch. 8(8.3)
19. False	Ch. 8(8.3)
20. False	Ch. 8(8.3)
21. False	Ch. 8(8.3)
22. True	Ch. 8(8.3)
23. B	Documented natural disease
24. A	Use of qualifiers acceptable
25. B	Ch. 8 (8.3)
26. C	Ch. 8(8.3)
27. C	Ch. 8(8.3)
28. A	Natural disease sequela with terminal fall

Appendix I
Part II: Self-Assessment: Death Certificate Critique Exercise
(answers appear at the end of this exercise)

For the following Cause and Manner-of-death statements, identify the error(s) present using the following lettered identifiers:

A: Incorrect sequencing or reversal of order of statements
B: Use of abbreviations and/or shorthand
C: Listing of more than one competing disease or disease condition per line
D: Sequential listing of causally unrelated diseases or disease conditions
E: Citing mechanisms, terminal events, and non-specific disease processes with omission of etiologic agent or etiologically specific underlying cause
F: Omission of descriptive characteristics of malignancy
G: Inclusion of injury or injury-associated complication in Part I or II with "Natural" listed as the manner of death
H. Reversal of Part I and Part II cause-of-death information

1.

Part I.	Approximate interval: Onset to death
A. **Hypotension**	**Days**
Due to (or as a consequence of): B.	
Due to (or as a consequence of): C.	
Due to (or as a consequence of): D.	
Part II. Other significant conditions contributing to death but not resulting in the underlying cause given in Part I	
	Manner of Death **Natural**

2.

Part I. A. **Cardiopulmonary arrest**	Approximate interval: Onset to death **Minutes**
Due to (or as a consequence of): B. **Sepsis**	**4 days**
Due to (or as a consequence of): C.	
Due to (or as a consequence of): D.	
Part II. Other significant conditions contributing to death but not resulting in the underlying cause given in Part I	
	Manner of Death **Natural**

3.

Part I. A. **Cardiac failure**	Approximate interval: Onset to death **6 hours**
Due to (or as a consequence of): B. **PE**	**12 hours**
Due to (or as a consequence of): C. **DVT**	**1 week**
Due to (or as a consequence of): D. **HCVD w/CHF**	**10 years**
Part II. Other significant conditions contributing to death but not resulting in the underlying cause given in Part I **NIDDM, S/P CABG X3, Rem. TAH**	
	Manner of Death **Natural**

4.

Part I. A. **Aortic atherosclerosis**	Approximate interval: Onset to death **10 Years**
Due to (or as a consequence of): B. **Abdominal aortic aneurysm with spontaneous acute rupture**	**5 years**
Due to (or as a consequence of): C. **Hemoperitoneum**	**6 hours**
Due to (or as a consequence of): D.	
Part II. Other significant conditions contributing to death but not resulting in the underlying cause given in Part I	
	Manner of Death **Natural**

5.

Part A. **Leg tumor**	Approximate interval: Onset to death **Months**
Due to (or as a consequence of): B.	
Due to (or as a consequence of): C.	
Due to (or as a consequence of): D.	
Part II. Other significant conditions contributing to death but not resulting in the underlying cause given in Part I	
	Manner of Death **Natural**

6.

Part I. A. **Hospital acquired pneumonia**	Approximate interval: Onset to death **< 1 week**
Due to (or as a consequence of): B. **C-6 quadriplegia**	**> 1 year**
Due to (or as a consequence of): C. **Mucous plugging**	**> 1 month**
Due to (or as a consequence of): D. **Heart failure**	**> 1 month**
Part II. Other significant conditions contributing to death but not resulting in the underlying cause given in Part I	
	Manner of Death **Natural**

7.

Part I. A. **Multisystem organ failure**	Approximate interval: Onset to death **1 week**
Due to (or as a consequence of): B. **Sepsis**	**2 weeks**
Due to (or as a consequence of): C. **Klebsiella pneumonia**	**3 weeks**
Due to (or as a consequence of): D.	
Part II. Other significant conditions contributing to death but not resulting in the underlying cause given in Part I **Paraplegia with multiple advanced decubital ulcers**	
	Manner of Death **Natural**

8.

Part I.	Approximate interval: Onset to death
A. **Cardiopulmonary arrest, Multiple Sclerosis Stage IV Advanced**	**Jan 2015**
Due to (or as a consequence of): B. **Sacral decubital ulcer, Neurogenic bladder**	**Years**
Due to (or as a consequence of): C. **Castrate resistant metastatic Ca prostate, quadriplegia**	**Years**
Due to (or as a consequence of): D. **Recurrent UTI**	**Years**
Part II. Other significant conditions contributing to death but not resulting in the underlying cause given in Part I	
	Manner of Death **Natural**

9.

Part I.	Approximate interval: Onset to death
A. **Cardiopulmonary arrest**	**1 day**
Due to (or as a consequence of): B.	
Due to (or as a consequence of): C.	
Due to (or as a consequence of): D.	
Part II. Other significant conditions contributing to death but not resulting in the underlying cause given in Part I **ESRD, S. Ulcer, HTN, Paraplegia**	
	Manner of Death **Natural**

10.

Part I. A. **Closed head injury**	Approximate interval: Onset to death **4 days**
Due to (or as a consequence of): B.	
Due to (or as a consequence of): C.	
Due to (or as a consequence of): D.	
Part II. Other significant conditions contributing to death but not resulting in the underlying cause given in Part I **Coronary artery disease, HCVD, DM**	
	Manner of Death **Natural**

11.

Part I. A. **Congestive heart failure**	Approximate interval: Onset to death **Days**
Due to (or as a consequence of): B. **Anemia**	**Months**
Due to (or as a consequence of): C. **Femur fracture**	**Weeks**
Due to (or as a consequence of): D. **COPD**	**Years**
Part II. Other significant conditions contributing to death but not resulting in the underlying cause given in Part I	
	Manner of Death **Natural**

12.

Part I.	Approximate interval: Onset to death
A. **Respiratory failure**	**Hours**
Due to (or as a consequence of): B. **Acute kidney injury**	**Days**
Due to (or as a consequence of): C. **Cholestasis**	**Weeks**
Due to (or as a consequence of): D. **Failure to thrive/debility**	**Months**
Part II. Other significant conditions contributing to death but not resulting in the underlying cause given in Part I	
	Manner of Death **Natural**

13.

Part I.	Approximate interval: Onset to death
A. **Cardiac arrest, CAD**	**1-2 hours**
Due to (or as a consequence of): B. **CAD, anemia, A-fib, intertrochanteric fracture**	**4-5 months**
Due to (or as a consequence of): C.	
Due to (or as a consequence of): D.	
Part II. Other significant conditions contributing to death but not resulting in the underlying cause given in Part I	
	Manner of Death **Natural**

14.

Part I.	Approximate interval: Onset to death
A. **Cardiopulmonary failure**	**1 day**
Due to (or as a consequence of): B. **Possible aspiration**	**1 day**
Due to (or as a consequence of): C. **Quadriparesis**	**Years**
Due to (or as a consequence of): D.	
Part II. Other significant conditions contributing to death but not resulting in the underlying cause given in Part I	
	Manner of Death **Natural**

15.

Part I.	Approximate interval: Onset to death
A. **Cardiopulmonary arrest**	**Minutes**
Due to (or as a consequence of): B. **Respiratory failure and hypoxia**	**Weeks**
Due to (or as a consequence of): C. **Bilateral pneumonia, ARDS, pul. fibrosis**	**Months**
Due to (or as a consequence of): D. **s/p fracture of hip and chr. dyspnea**	**Months**
Part II. Other significant conditions contributing to death but not resulting in the underlying cause given in Part I	
	Manner of Death **Natural**

16.

Part I. A. **Obesity**	Approximate interval: Onset to death **Years**
Due to (or as a consequence of): B.	
Due to (or as a consequence of): C.	
Due to (or as a consequence of): D.	
Part II. Other significant conditions contributing to death but not resulting in the underlying cause given in Part I **Non-alcoholic steatohepatitis, hepatic cirrhosis, hepatic encephalopathy**	
	Manner of Death **Natural**

Part II: Self-Assessment/Death Certificate Critique Exercise-Answers

1. E
2. E
3. B
4. A
5. F
6. B, D, E, G (errors also prompt entry of illogical, non-progressive onset-to-death time intervals)
7. G
8. B, C, D, G
9. B, E, G
10. B, G
11. B, D, G
12. C, D, G
13. B, C, G (CAD is also repeated on line B)
14. E, G
15. B, C, D, G
16. H

INDEX

A

B

C

D

E

F

G

H

I

M

N

O

P

Q

R

S

T

U

V

W

www.ingramcontent.com/pod-product-compliance
Lightning Source LLC
Chambersburg PA
CBHW080529220326
41599CB00032B/6254